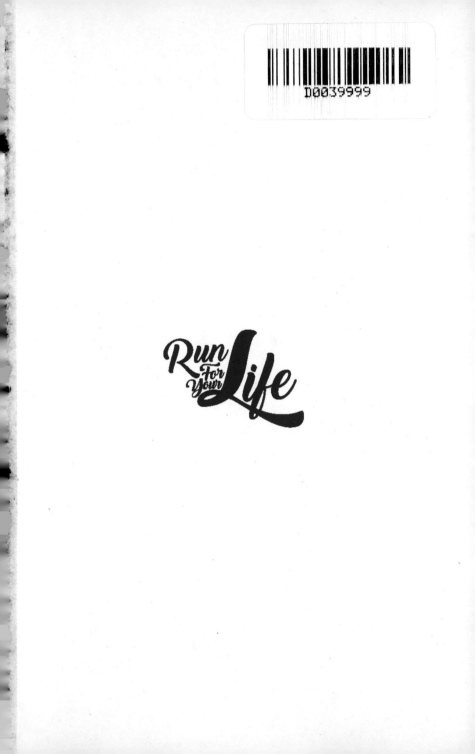

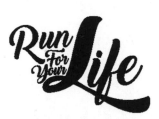

HOW ONE WOMAN
RAN CIRCLES AROUND
BREAST CANCER

JENNY BAKER

First published by Pitch Publishing, 2017

Pitch Publishing
A2 Yeoman Gate
Yeoman Way
Worthing
Sussex
BN13 3QZ

www.pitchpublishing.co.uk
info@pitchpublishing.co.uk

A CIP catalogue record is available for this book
from the British Library.

ISBN 978-1-78531-261-8

Typesetting and origination by Pitch Publishing
Printed by 4edge Limited, Essex, UK

Contents

For my chemo runners

*Lucy, Harry, Chris, Mandy,
Liz, Joel and Neil
and for Jonny, always*

1

The Best-Laid Plans...

I FIND the last long run before a marathon comes with a huge sense of relief. It is the sign that the bulk of your training is over; you can do no more to influence your performance on the day except sleep, eat well and try not to trip up kerbs. I know lots of runners struggle with the taper at the end of a training plan, the couple of weeks when you reduce the mileage so you can start the race on rested legs, but actually I like that shift in gear, from investing in training to needing to trust it.

Inevitably you wonder if you have done enough and whether you will be able to deliver on race day, but over the next couple of weeks there is a growing sense of anticipation at being about to find out what you are capable of.

This particular last long run had added significance for me because this was the first time I was going to do two marathons in close succession – the Palestine Marathon in Bethlehem at the end of March followed by London a month later. I learned from my 40th that significant birthdays pass better when they are significantly celebrated, so as well as parties with friends and family I had decided to mark turning 50 in 2015 by doing what I loved most: running.

Secretly I wanted to do five marathons that year – Palestine, London, Bath in the autumn with my sister, my first 50km ultra along the Suffolk coast and another one somewhere in between just because I could – although I had not yet admitted to all of those out loud. The previous year had been my best year of running; I had got a PB in every distance I had run and had done my highest annual mileage ever. I felt happier in my skin approaching my 50th birthday than at any other time in my life, and running was a huge contributing factor, giving me a sense of physical, spiritual and mental well-being. Life was good.

My plan on that cold day in March was to do a 20-mile loop, running along roads through Kew to Richmond, following the trail inside the perimeter of Richmond Park and then home along the river with a lap of Ealing Common at the end to make up the distance. Urban runners need to be more intentional about finding green spaces and trails to run in, and this route had a good mix of scenery and surfaces. It also had a reasonable number of inclines, which are few and far between in Ealing where I live. Palestine is a hilly marathon, run over a two-lap course because there are not 26.2 consecutive miles on the roads leading out of Bethlehem without checkpoints on the way. It is a tough course because although more people take part each year, not many do the full marathon and you end up running most of it on your own which is why I was doing this training run solo.

Having made it up the long slow rise of Richmond Hill and past the old Royal Star and Garter Home for injured servicemen that was now being turned into luxury flats, it was a relief to turn in to the park and follow the trail round the edge. Richmond Park is the closest we west-Londoners can get to proper countryside, created 400 years earlier as a hunting park for royalty. It has areas of wide-open scrublands filled with ancient trees where deer still roam as well as ponds, rugby pitches and woodland gardens. It is a busy place, a magnet for cyclists and runners and a scenic cut-through for cars on their way to south London. But it is one of my favourite places to run, a place to breathe deeply and savour the trails, a place to forget the urban sprawl that lies on the other side of the wall and try to spot the deer under the trees. I settled into a steady pace after the exertion of the hill, running on autopilot.

And then, all at once:

a tug as my foot catches on something;
confusion as the ground rushes to meet me;
a futile attempt to break my fall with my hands;
an involuntary grunt as the breath is knocked from me;
a thud as my knee hits the ground and a smack as my
cheekbone lands on tarmac.
Split-second silence.
Stillness.

Shakily, I get up and hobble back to the path. It takes me a little while to work out what has happened and what to do next. I had tripped on something and landed on the road across the entrance to the car park. My leggings had ripped and my knee was bleeding. I could feel that my lip was already starting to swell. I made my way over to the café and asked to use their toilets.

Disinterested, the guy behind the counter waved me over to the portakabins at the far side of the car park. There were other people around, runners, cyclists and dog walkers but no one stopped to ask me how I was or find out whether they could help. I assessed the damage in the mirror, dabbing at my face with some damp loo paper and cursing my lack of attention that had led to my fall. What should I do? I could ring Jonny, my husband, to get him to come and pick me up, or keep going and do the route that I had planned.

I decided on a middle option, to run back home from there; it wouldn't be quite the 20 miles in my schedule but it would be closer than the nine that I had just done. My knee felt stiff as I set off but after a while it loosened up a bit and I plodded for home.

Five miles later I had to admit defeat. My knee was really painful. I had almost reached Kew Bridge, which is a couple of miles from my home. I got my phone out and pressed Jonny's name to call him, only for the wheel of death to appear on the screen and for the battery to die. I allowed myself some tears of self-pity as I realised my only option was to walk.

It takes a moment to trip; it takes longer to realise the full implications. Two hours later, I was eating breakfast in the kitchen after a shower, feeling more positive now I was warm again and determined that this was not going to derail my plans. Three days later I was tired of having to explain where my marvellous black eye had come from and was trying to be patient about getting back to running. A week later, I tried a tentative couple of miles round the common only to realise that this was more serious than I thought.

After several trips to the physio, I had to admit I wasn't going to run a marathon in Palestine and I withdrew from London as well, devastated that everything was going wrong. Of course I *knew* that there would be other races, that I would recover from my injuries, that it wasn't the end of the world, but what I *felt* was a visceral sense of loss, a death of a dream and a fear that this could be the end of my running.

In March, I went to Palestine but just ran the 10k because my knee couldn't take any more. And in April I watched my son and my friends do the London Marathon, loving the occasion and enjoying their achievements. In between the two, I had found out that a couple of missed races was trivial compared to the challenge that lay ahead. That fall in the park was just the start of this year not turning out as I planned.

2

Becoming a Runner

I CAN tell you when I became a mother, when I became a teacher, when I became a mother-in-law. The memories of where these shifts in identity took place are strong – giving birth, my first job, my son's wedding. It is harder to pinpoint when I became a runner, that moment when running changed from being something that I occasionally did in my spare time, to being a core strand of my identity.

But I can remember my first race. Jonny and I moved to London when we were both 30, with our two young sons Joel and Harry, who were five and three respectively. We had lived in Bath before that and discovered when we turned up in Ealing that lots of parents we met aspired to do the opposite, to move out of the urban sprawl to somewhere 'safe' and 'beautiful' for their children to grow up.

Like many women my age I was juggling work and parenting, and struggling to make friends in this rather bewildering city. I joined the local YMCA gym and one of the trainers there encouraged me to do a 5k race they were putting on in the local park.

My memory is hazy about how much training I did, but I remember going out to run round the park in preparation. On the day, there was a group of proper runners who filled the space near the start line with their club running shirts and their confident talk about other races they had done.

I hung back, feeling like a fraud, but when the race began I found myself drawn into their orbit, trying to keep up. Having set off far too fast, it wasn't long before I had to walk to try and get my breathing back under control. The rest of the race went the same way, spurts of trying to run properly interwoven with bouts of embarrassed walking. It was not a huge success. I have no record of my time, of whether there was a medal, or of where I finished in the standings but I can still conjure up that feeling of not fitting in, of not being a 'proper' runner.

A couple of years later, I was working for a charity when one of my colleagues, Lorna, got a corporate entry into the second year of the London Triathlon. She and her husband were keen to do it as a personal challenge but also to raise money for the charity. What she perhaps had not thought through was the fact that most other people working there were far from sporty and her increasingly desperate requests for people who would use the other three entries eventually wore me down. I said I would have a go. Jonny's response, not surprisingly given my underwhelming 5k performance, was to laugh at me but that only made me more determined.

We signed up for the Olympic distance, a 1,500m swim in open water, a 40k cycle and a 10k run. I had never done those distances in any of the three disciplines before. I went to the pool more often in preparation and cycled when I could, as well as running a couple of times a week. Not a very effective training plan, I now realise, but that was all I knew. I bought an occasional copy of a triathlon magazine, but found its advice complex and intimidating.

The day before the race, I took my bike over to the Excel Centre in the London Docklands, and left it on a crowded rack in a vast hall, its bulky lime-green frame and mountain bike tyres standing out like a sore thumb among the sleek and skinny machines that everyone else seemed to have. Race day was grey and cold, and as my wave made our way down to the water's edge, we passed an ambulance with a group of people crowded round someone who had just been fished out of the water. My stomach was a churning mass of nerves, but it was only when the swim started that the enormity of what I was attempting truly hit me and I realised how poor my preparation had been.

It seems incredible to me now, but my first ever experience of open-water swimming was during this open-water race. I had done several sessions in my hired wetsuit at the local pool during my training but just hadn't appreciated how different it is to swim in a lake, or river or dock compared to swimming in a leisure centre. There is no blue row of tiles on the floor making sure you swim in a straight line. There is no floor, at least not one that you can see, just a murky greenness when you put your head in the water.

The start was a mass of thrashing arms and legs as the swim got underway but it was not long before I was left in a scary calm as everyone else surged ahead. I felt completely overwhelmed and came very close to abandoning the race at the start, but the thought of having to admit to the 60 or so people who had sponsored me to do this that I had given up kept me going. I did the whole 1,500m in breaststroke with my head out of the water, painfully slowly. Towards the end, I waved to my family who were patiently standing on the edge of a dock, and a safety marshal in a kayak zoomed over to check I was okay. I had inadvertently used the distress signal when all I wanted to communicate was that I was still alive and persevering. As tempting as it was to seek refuge on his boat, I kept going.

Finally, finally I made it to the end where another couple of marshals helped me out of the water and on to my feet. My legs gave way as I tried to stand and one of them helpfully said, 'You can do a sprint distance, you know.'

The rest of the race was a blur. According to the results that I faithfully recorded in a spreadsheet, I spent nearly two hours on my mountain bike, most of it being overtaken by people who started in the wave behind me. Proper triathletes practise their transitions to minimise the time spent going from one discipline to the next. I went to the loo after I got off my bike, to try and delay the moment when I had to start running.

The three laps of the run each seemed far longer than the one before and all contained a fair amount of walking, but I finally turned the corner into the finishing stretch to see Lorna and my poor long-suffering family still standing there to cheer me on. 'Look at the time, Jenny,' Lorna shouted to me but I had no idea what she meant.

I stumbled to the finishing line, overwhelmed with relief that now I could finally stop running. My time was 4 hours and 24 seconds; Lorna had been trying to encourage me to come in under four hours but I had no reserves of energy to draw from to turn my stagger into a run. Still, I had done my first triathlon.

And I had got the bug. In the weeks that followed, I realised how much I had loved setting myself this challenge and rising to it. I loved being fit and I loved the regular discipline of exercise so I continued to do Olympic-distance triathlons over the next ten years, slowly improving on my time and technique. I invested many hours and lots of money into learning to swim front crawl over a period of four years, working my way through a friend who offered to coach me, a class at my local swimming pool, and an intensive weekend course whose hosts assured me it was suitable for beginners. It was not.

In the end, I paid a private swimming coach an extortionate amount of money to work with me one-to-one and it was worth it. The first time I swam 60 lengths of a pool non-stop, the magical 1,500m I would need to do in a triathlon, I burst into tears at the end much to the consternation of the guy next to me who gave me a worried look and quickly dived under water.

It is often said that running is the cheapest and easiest form of exercise, and at one level that is true. You just put on your trainers and get out the front door. Inevitably though, the longer you do it the more professionals and the more products get drawn into becoming an essential part of your experience.

I went to see a physio while I was training for triathlons because I couldn't run far without my knee hurting. I now know that was my ITB band protesting and what was needed was regular time with a foam roller. He talked me into an expensive habit of treatments with ultrasound and didn't once show me the stretches that would have solved the problem. Fortunately charlatans like him are few and far between, and if I had had some running companions they would have alerted me sooner that I was wasting my cash.

I also had regular problems with my lower back giving way. I sought out a chiropractor after I pulled a muscle in my back just reaching for the shampoo in the shower, and she diagnosed a wonky pelvis that she gradually got back into alignment for me. My running experience was transformed. My knee stopped hurting, I could run further and more freely and could expect my body to deliver more when I asked it to.

A friend, Kevin Draper, had a go at triathlons after he saw my first London experience and had an even stronger conversion than me. His investment in training saw him competing impressively at age-group standard and he qualified as a coach. He offered to coach me for what would be my final triathlon in 2008, although I didn't realise it at the time, and I finished in less than three hours, an improvement on my original time that I was really pleased with.

But training for three sports takes hours each week; I would swim twice, run twice and try to fit in a long cycle. When I started a Masters degree in gender studies in my spare time the following autumn, I realised how precious that spare time was. I had to admit to my competitive self that if I did another triathlon I would want to better my time, but what with work, parenting and study I just didn't currently have the spare hours I needed to invest in training.

But I also knew that I needed to keep doing some kind of exercise. I had been introduced to the Ignatian examen, a regular practice of reflecting on the events of the day and identifying the moments that give life and those that drain energy. It was developed by St Ignatius, the Spanish founder of the Jesuits, while he was recovering from terrible injuries suffered in a battle against the French. Through long static days in bed, he recognised that some of his thoughts and daydreams left him downhearted and deadened, while others left him energised and excited about the future. He crafted this insight into the examen, a practice of looking back on your day and asking 'for what moment am I most grateful?', and then 'for what moment am I least grateful?' Over time the answers to these questions help you discern where God might be active in your life and what you might be called to.

The idea is that you can learn from both consolation and desolation, that each is an invitation to growth. You can choose to make space in your life for more of the things that cause gratitude and pay attention to what drains life from you.

Over a period of time I recognised that running and exercise were the things I was most grateful for. I felt guilty at first, feeling that I ought to have identified something more spiritual, that surely running could not count. But the more I thought about it, the more I realised how much running meant to me and how much it contributed to my well-being, physically, mentally and spiritually, so running became an essential part of my life and in 2009 I set myself a different kind of challenge, a half-marathon.

Every race starts with some kind of question. Can I run this far? Can I run that fast? Have I done enough training? What difference does this cold make? Is my knee fixed? Am I faster than her yet? And you only find the answer by running the race. I signed up for the Folkestone Half-Marathon wondering if I could run that far and discovered that I could. Each race not only answers a question, it also sets another target, a time to beat or a training plan to improve or a different course to conquer. I finished Folkestone in just under two hours and wondered how much faster I could go.

And I also wondered how much further I could run. When I did triathlons, people would often ask me if I was going to run a marathon and I always said no because of the problems I had with my knee. A 10k had seemed to be my running limit. But now my chiropractor had straightened me out, now I had done a half-marathon, maybe a marathon was not impossible.

One day I spent time with Letty Wilson, a friend who I had known from university. We had done a maths and computing degree together, had briefly become maths teachers and had been each other's best women when we got married. Although we now lived 30 miles apart, we still made the effort to see each other regularly. By now we were both in our mid-40s and she started talking about the things she hoped to achieve by the time she was 50. I had not particularly thought about getting that old yet, but I was struck by one of the things on her list – running a marathon. I borrowed the idea from her and looked around for one to sign up to.

What exactly is it that spurs us on to go further or to be faster? For me it was the new horizon that was opened up by each achievement. I had been painfully shy as a teenager and although I had overcome much of that as I had grown up, I had always had a loud internal voice criticising what I was doing and keeping me in check. Achieving the challenges of doing a triathlon, conquering front crawl, running my first half-marathon all helped me see myself in a new light even though I was hesitant to own the labels in public, as a triathlete, a swimmer, and a runner. If I could do these things that I had once thought impossible, what else was within my reach? What else could I achieve if I only tried?

I was still very much a solo runner trying to work it out for myself. Knowing nothing about marathons, I looked online for one to enter. It was towards the end of the year and most of the marathons I found via the Runner's World website were already full so I entered the first one near me that still had spaces, the inaugural Sussex Marathon in April 2011, and signed up for their training plan. When you know very little about something, you put yourself in the hands of those who seem to have the expertise you are lacking.

The training plan was three runs a week, gradually extending the long run towards 20 miles. I still felt on the outside of this world of running, and lacked the confidence to interrogate it and make it my own. So I just faithfully followed the plan, building up the mileage and logging it on a spreadsheet when I got home. I remember the first time I ran 16 miles and arrived back exhausted, wondering how on earth I would ever manage another ten miles on top of that. But the plan for the next week said 18 miles, so that is what I did and gradually built up to 22 miles which made me feel perhaps I could run a marathon after all.

The race organisers had to alter the route they had advertised because they didn't get permission to close the roads. Instead of the meandering course through country roads that they had aspired to, the route ended up being a six-mile loop starting in Battle, and then an out-and-back hilly run to Ashburnham that you had to do twice. The race fell on Mothers' Day, so Jonny and I invited his mum, Alison, who lived nearby in Sussex, to come and watch the race with him while I ran – how generous of us!

I felt incredibly nervous before the start, and got very, very cold. I started the race wearing a jacket with my race number pinned on the front and with pockets full of energy gels to keep me going through several hours of running. My target time was 4 hours 20 minutes and I set off at a steady pace, determined not to repeat my 5k mistake by starting too fast too soon.

Of course as I got going, I warmed up and then overheated. Mile five was spent unpinning my race number from my jacket and replacing it on my top underneath while still running, then fishing out the gels from the pockets and squirrelling them away on my body – a couple tucked under my bra straps, two more stuffed down the front of my leggings. When I passed Jonny and his mum in Battle at the end of the first loop, I thrust my jacket into their outstretched arms and continued down the road, trying to stop a gel from migrating down the inside of my leggings to my feet, while still running. I think I ended up trapping it in my knickers.

In my memory, the trek to Ashburnham is like a sine wave, one vicious hill after another with the downhills in between giving a meagre feeling of respite. I managed to run the first 18 miles of the race, but the next hill defeated me and I had to walk. And once I had walked once it was impossible not to do it again. The last eight miles of my race turned into a laboured walk up one hill and an unsteady jog down to the next. My target time came and went and disappeared into the ether. I finished the race in 5 hours and 3 minutes, aware in the last few miles that I would be close to the magical five-hour target but, like my triathlon experience, unable to summon any extra energy to hit it.

I collected my medal just after crossing the line and went to meet my very bored husband and his mum. I felt wobbly and emotional, and strangely disappointed that it had been so hard and had taken me so long. I didn't have much of a sense of achievement. I thought I had done enough training in preparation, but I had underestimated just how much a marathon takes out of you physically, mentally and emotionally. If I were ever to do another one, I would need a different approach.

That summer a message arrived via Facebook from Godfrey Rust, a friend whose son had been in the same class as Harry at school. 'Hi Jenny – just remembered you're a regular runner. A couple of months ago I joined Ealing Eagles, who do park runs in our territory on Monday and Wednesday evenings – good fun sociable crowd, all standards and ages, equal split male/female. Thought I'd mention it in case it would fit your schedule to run with a bunch of others anytime. It's helping me in my struggle to get back to some kind of fitness!'

So began a whole new chapter of my running life and I joined the Ealing Eagles Running Club in July 2011. It took me a while to get into it. The first few runs I turned up for, I felt awkward and didn't really talk to anyone. But the more runs I went to, the more I began to feel I belonged. The active Facebook group for the club made it easier to get to know people and remember names. I made friends and started to work out who was a similar runner to me. And best of all, I got to know Kelvin Walker, who was training to be a running coach and needed someone to practise on.

Kelvin is an accountant by training and someone who throws himself fully into whatever is in front of him. As well as doing his coaching training, he was the Eagles' treasurer, he led the beginners' sessions for the club, and he was hatching a plan with some others to set up a half-marathon in Ealing the following autumn. Kelvin is a wonderfully positive person, a natural encourager, and he does a mean Bruce Springsteen impression after a few pints of beer.

I had decided that I wanted to try another marathon so had signed up for Brighton in April 2012, and Kelvin kindly agreed to coach me for it. He designed a training plan for me and we met weekly to talk about how things were going. I had done a few more half-marathons by then, and based on those times, I decided to aim for a sub-four-hour marathon at Brighton. Kelvin encouraged me to have more than one goal for the race, so that whatever time I did it in there would be something to celebrate. My first goal was to run all the way as I had walked some of the previous marathon; the next to beat my time from the year before; then to shave an hour off my PB; and then the top goal, to finish in under four hours.

The encouragement and wisdom of a coach and the friendship and healthy competition of other runners made all the difference to my training experience. One Sunday that winter I woke up to snow on the ground. I had been planning to do the club ten-mile run that morning and checked the website to find that it was officially cancelled for safety reasons, but I was sure that wouldn't put everyone off.

I went downstairs in my running kit, to the ridicule of my family who thought snow was the best excuse to spend the morning in bed. I made my way up to the club run meeting point on Ealing Green to find another dozen runners there, and we set off in high spirits for our unofficial run, not worried about speed, but just enjoying the beauty and playfulness of running in snow. My heart was full as I ran; these were people for whom running marathons was normal, who were not put off by a bit of snow, who got why running was worth pursuing. This was my tribe.

Training with Kelvin's input felt much more purposeful and enlightened. My training had more variety and I understood why each of the different sessions in the week was important. I relished the challenge of the 16-week plan I was following, and really appreciated having such an encouraging and positive coach. But the disappointment of the year before nagged at me. I found myself thinking after each session, 'Well I've managed that one, but I don't know if I'll be able to do the next.'

And then one day it clicked. Marathon training is an act of faith. The running that I had already done had set me up for the running that I was going to do in the future; I will be able to run tomorrow because I ran yesterday. I started approaching my next sessions, not with the dread that I would fail, but with a curiosity to discover what my body could now do. You run with your whole being, not just your legs, and that means your mind and your spirit too.

Over the years I have found the most difficult aspect of running is training my mind, developing that mental endurance that enables me to keep going when everything in me says stop. I realised that that is where I needed to trust the training I have done, the wisdom and experience behind the training plans I have followed, the encouragement and support of friends who have run more marathons than me, the belief of a coach who could see the potential that I doubted, the memories of the winter runs in the dark and the snow which had set me up for my Brighton race.

I ended up going down to Brighton on my own. Jonny had little interest in running and had no wish to repeat the tedium of the previous year's spectating experience, and I didn't know anyone else in the club who was doing the race. Kelvin had the final session of his coaching course that day so couldn't be there to cheer me on.

I stayed with friends in Brighton the night before, who fed me pasta and gave me a lift to the start. This time my nerves were more manageable, a gentle reminder that this was a serious undertaking but one that was within my grasp. It was a much larger race than Sussex with thousands of entrants rather than hundreds, and the start of the race was really crowded. I struggled to get into my groove as I weaved through other runners and did my second and third miles far too fast. But then my race head kicked in, the other runners thinned out and I settled into a steady pace.

The Brighton Marathon starts inland at Preston Park but most of it is run along the coast. It was a bright, sunny day and the sparkling sea was a fantastic backdrop to the determined efforts of the runners. I find races inspiring, to think of all the time and effort that has gone into training, the goals and dreams that runners are pursuing, the different things that have motivated people to enter this race. It is very moving seeing people running in charity shirts or with people's faces or names on their backs, a story of loss or challenge behind each runner.

I was running with my dad in mind. He had been growing increasingly frail over the previous couple of years and was now confined to bed. He had been a talented runner when he was young, and had won cross-country, 800m and 1,500m British Army championships when he had done his National Service. I had been to see him a couple of weeks before the marathon and had talked to him about the race. He said 'run it for me' so I had ironed the words 'For my Dad' on to the back of my shirt.

The attraction of the sea view began to pale towards the end of the race. From mile 19 the course heads out towards the power station by Shoreham Harbour, an industrial area with few spectators, and I found the next few miles a hard slog. I was wearing a pace band with the mile splits for a four-hour race, and had been watching my Garmin GPS watch closely, which told me how far and how fast I was going. The mental calculations of what pace I needed to do to hit my target were a welcome distraction from the pain in my legs. I could see that if I kept going at my current pace I was likely to finish in just over four hours, but even though I tried to speed up and I felt like I was putting more effort in, my watch showed me the unwelcome truth that I was actually getting slower.

Sure enough, I finished in 4 hours and 2 minutes. Those first post-race minutes, when you have finally stopped running, bring an intense exhaustion. Initially I felt some disappointment not to have gone under four hours, but then I realised I had hit three out of my four targets. It is not bad to do your second marathon over an hour faster than your first, and it showed how much better my training had been thanks to the coaching I had had from Kelvin. I texted him and my dad with my time, and made my weary way home, delighted with what I had achieved.

Later that year I did my Leader in Running Fitness qualification with Mark Yabsley, a basic one-day coaching course that qualifies you to lead a running group. Mark gave me a lift to where the course was being held in Teddington, and we swapped stories about our running experiences on the way over. Mark had had an episode of ME many years before which had prompted him to rethink his career and retrain, and he now ran his own gardening business.

Mark and I joined Kelvin's beginners' course as volunteers and soon took over leading it. It was a six-week course that got people doing the local parkrun, a free, timed 5k race that happened in nearby Gunnersbury Park. The first session started with running for two minutes, then walking for two, repeated several times. Some people struggled to do that at first and for them, the goal of being able to run continuously for 5k seemed out of reach. I loved watching people progress from week to week, seeing their confidence grow and their fitness improve. It was a joy to do the parkrun with them at the end of the six weeks, to see them achieve the goal that had felt unattainable just a few weeks before.

I found it interesting that almost all of the people who came to our beginners' group were female, while there was a much more even split of men and women in the actual club. That kind of imbalance always makes me ask why it is happening. It seemed that most men got themselves into running and didn't feel the need of a structured course to help them.

We encouraged people to talk during the beginners' group; it is a good way of ensuring you set out at the right kind of pace because if you can't hold a conversation while you are running then you are definitely going too fast. Chatting to women as we ran about why they had joined, it was clear that there were a variety of reasons, because, after all, women are very diverse; we are not carbon copies of each other. Some didn't have the confidence to just turn up to a club run. Some hadn't done any exercise since school and needed the accountability and motivation of a structured plan. Some wanted to get to know other runners and figured, rightly, that the beginners' group was a good way of connecting with people. And some women were afraid to run on their own, feeling that the streets were too risky, particularly in the dark, and they wanted the safety of numbers.

I could identify with that last reason because I had often wrestled with the same issue as I decided where and when I would run over the years. The reality is that women grow up with the threat of attack and rape by strangers, and that fear restricts our movement. It stops us going out late or on our own, makes us hyper-alert when we are in a secluded area, and puts some places completely out of bounds to us.

But it is important to get the risk in perspective. Crime figures show that it is men who are more likely to be on the receiving end of a violent attack by a stranger and most rapes are perpetrated by someone known to those attacked. Every woman will have to make her own choice about what she is comfortable with. As I thought about where it was safe to run, I did not want to be naïve or unwise, but nor did I want to collude with that climate of fear and let it dictate how I moved around when actually the risk is pretty small.

In fact, in over 15 years of running I had only had two encounters that had made me feel uncomfortable and made me question the safety of running. One Sunday morning I went out quite early and was running along the river from Richmond to Kew on my way home. Ahead of me, I could see a man in the distance, crouching by the path and pointing his hand towards me as if it was a gun. As I got nearer, he slunk across the path in front of me to crouch on the opposite side, keeping his finger trained on me as I ran past.

My initial reaction was one of fear – what was he doing? Was he going to come after me? I couldn't see anyone else in front of me and when I looked back he had disappeared, but that meant I didn't know where he was.

I was relieved to see some other runners and a cyclist approaching and kept glancing back to check I was not being followed. It unsettled me but once I was safely back home I got really angry. This man had encroached on my run, on what I thought of as my space, and had made me feel unsafe doing something that I loved.

The other encounter happened at the end of a run after I had bought a newspaper and breakfast pastries at the local shop. As I walked back across the common, a guy who was completely high on something walked alongside me, chatting and telling me how fit my legs were. There were people around in the distance but I was going back to an empty house and I obviously did not want him to know where I lived.

As we got closer to the end of my road I had to tell him very strongly to stop following me. He eventually complied and he was so off his head I suspect he wouldn't have any memory of it later, but I did feel wary the next few times I went out running 'just in case' he was around.

Both of those incidents stayed with me for a while and had an impact on where I felt safe, but two unsettling encounters in thousands of runs in 15 years, neither of which harmed me at all, is a fairly insignificant threat. I was glad that our beginners' group was a way for women to address that fear, and I hoped that it would help them get the risk in perspective so that their freedom was not curtailed unnecessarily.

So where in that litany of running experiences did I become a runner? Actually, I think anyone who runs can call themselves a runner. You don't need to run far or run fast, to have done a certain number of races or conquered a particular distance. I was a runner after that first 5k. I need not have felt intimidated by the running club shirts and I am sure the people wearing them wouldn't have wanted me to. I had as much right to be there as anyone else. But I think I most *felt* like a runner after I had joined the Eagles, when I became part of a community of runners who shared my love of running and spurred each other on to new challenges.

Running was by now a regular habit. It was my headspace and a huge source of well-being, mentally, physically and emotionally. Running had given me a new community to belong to, and a new skill to use in the coaching I was doing for beginners. But running could be a whole lot more. The year after I did Brighton, I discovered running as an expression of a basic human right, running as a form of protest and running as an act of solidarity with people whose freedom was limited but whose spirits remained strong. I went running in Palestine.

3

Running in Palestine

WE are standing in front of an eight-metre-high concrete wall. Its ugliness is in sharp contrast to the abundant sunshine and bright blue sky of this day. Its height means we have to crane our necks to see the top. Its presence is a deep affront to the welcome we have found, a jarring disruption to travelling around this place, a very physical reminder of who has power around here. Graffiti words of protest and defiance cover the concrete, testament to the strong feelings people have about it but also their powerlessness to change it; it needs much more than slogans to dismantle this wall.

I am struggling to get my head round how people live in its shadow without going mad. And it throws a long shadow, both physical and psychological, dominating the landscape and the conversation, in front of people's faces and inside their heads. Getting ready to come here, I had read up on some of the history of this place, and deflected concerns from family and friends about whether it was safe to travel. I had packed sunscreen and my running gear, but nothing had prepared me for the visceral sense of injustice I feel walking round this place, that mix of incredulity and anger that asks how can this be allowed to happen?

It is 2012 and I am in Bethlehem in the West Bank with a group of artists. Since 1948, Palestine has been made up of two separate areas of land, the Gaza Strip on the coast of the Mediterranean Sea, and the West Bank about 40 miles away inland, so named because it lies to the west of the River Jordan. In between the two is the state of Israel.

I am on a trip organised by Greenbelt Arts Festival, taking people from different creative disciplines to experience something of what life is like in Palestine. For the previous two years I had been acting director of Greenbelt, and I had been given a place on this trip as a leaving present. There is a painter, a novelist, a filmmaker, an actor, a poet, a writer, a musician, several activists and me. The leader of our trip is Chris Rose, the director of Amos Trust, a creative human rights charity.

Chris is tall and gangly, not unlike Roald Dahl's Big Friendly Giant, with a restless energy and a passion for this land and its people. As we travel around, he gives us the background to the places we are visiting and explains some of the issues that make living here difficult, patiently answering our questions and making sure we have understood. He makes the bus driver stop by the side of the road so we can drink real Arabic coffee from a street seller, and tells us how we can recognise Palestinian homes as we drive by; they are the ones with the black water tanks on the roof because their access to water is so limited.

It is easier not to voice an opinion on what is happening in this part of the Middle East. The history of Israel/Palestine is long and complicated, and many different nations have wrestled over control of this land through the centuries. Any explanation quickly becomes a history lesson, with the dates of what happened when peppered through it, and there are many different ways to tell the story of the same set of events. The atrocities inflicted on the Jewish people over centuries are the back story to this episode of course, and the context in which any discussion about Israel/Palestine takes place.

History tells us that its all too easy for the oppressed to become the oppressor, but when any critique of the Israeli government is met with cries of anti-Semitism it can be hard to raise awareness of how Palestinians are suffering disproportionately under the occupation. Although the history of this place is complex, the main issue is really quite simple. There should be full equal rights for everyone who calls the historic land of Palestine home. Many books have been written about what is going on here; all I can tell you is what I am seeing and hearing.

Walls are built in the name of security, but Bethlehem shows that this wall is not only about security. We walk along its route from the checkpoint leading into the town, to where it crosses what used to be the main road to Hebron. Along the way it snakes around three sides of a house, surrounding it in concrete, cutting it off from its neighbours.

The owner of the house, Claire, comes out to tell us how the wall went up in a day. Her English is impeccable and her hazel eyes hold ours as she recounts what happened. She tells this story to everyone who walks past, desperate for her family's experience to be heard, for the injustice of it to be acknowledged. Her children went to school in the morning and came back to find their house isolated by concrete, the view from their bedroom windows cut off; her seven-year-old son cries that he feels like he is being buried in a tomb. The thriving gift shop on the ground floor of their house is now moribund; few people come down here any more now that it is a dead end.

The reason the wall detours round Claire's house is because on the other side of it is Rachel's Tomb, a holy site for Jewish people, along with a coach park and an army outpost. Israelis and tourists can now travel from Jerusalem to the Tomb without going into Bethlehem; Palestinians cannot visit it at all. This wall separates Palestinian from Palestinian; it cuts off farmers from their land; it disrupts children's journeys to school and their parents' travel to work.

Meg Wroe, the artist in our group, goes into a local school to get children creating artwork. She has brought paintings from a London school that she works in, and messages from the pupils there for their peers in Bethlehem. The children draw pictures of themselves for Meg to take back with her. The local teacher is delighted with what they produce, and the excitement it generates.

She tells Meg, 'Once they are about ten years old, all they will draw is the wall.'

We visit Al-Walaja, a beautiful village just outside Bethlehem, surrounded by ancient olive groves. Much of Al-Walaja is in Area C, the part of Palestine that is under Israeli civil administration and security control. Palestinian families have lived here for generations, the land passed down from father to son, over and over again. But although people own their land, it is very difficult to get permission from the Israeli government to build on it. People build anyway. Families expand, and each new generation needs somewhere to live, so they squeeze new homes in between the houses that are already there; there is nowhere else to go. Demolition orders get served on houses built without permission, and homes are demolished with little warning.

The year before, Chris had brought a team of people over to Al-Walaja to rebuild a home that had been bulldozed. People from the UK raised money for the materials and to pay professional builders, and then came to do the unskilled labour of moving bricks and buckets of cement. Over 200 homes were demolished in 2011 in Gaza and the West Bank, making over 1,000 Palestinians homeless; rebuilding one house is a drop in the ocean, but it is also an audacious statement of solidarity and resistance. A few weeks after the team left, a new demolition order was served on the house, the family's joy at their new home once again tainted with the uncertainty of how long it will last.

We visit the family and listen to their story. We drink Arabic coffee in their garden, and walk down the valley with their young daughter to touch the centuries-old olive trees that have seen conflicts come and go, wondering how such inhumanity can take root in such a beautiful place.

Back in Bethlehem, we walk through Aida Refugee Camp, a dense and sprawling cluster of buildings that has been home to refugees since 1950. The UN is responsible here. Unemployment and frustration are high; resources and expectation are low. We meet Mohammed, a student in his early twenties who, like everyone around here, is happy to talk to us and tell us his story. He wants to be a human rights lawyer. He was enrolled in a university in Jerusalem, but the difficulty of the journey has made it too hard to keep up with his studies. Jerusalem is less than ten kilometres from here, less than an hour's run, but there are checkpoints between here and there with unpredictable waits and too frequent restrictions on travel. Mohammed has had to accept the narrowing of his horizons and has changed courses to study here in Bethlehem. He knows that his qualification will not be recognised in Israel, his options will be fewer. I realise that Mohammed is the same age as my son Joel who is studying art back in London and has the world at his feet, and the contrast seems so unfair.

While I fight back tears, I hear Chris ask him, 'Barcelona or Madrid?' It is the international language of football. They get into an animated discussion about the merits of their respective teams. They are no longer refugee and privileged Westerner, just two fans exchanging banter and insults. Normally, I have an inbuilt aversion to professional football. I think it promotes a particularly toxic form of masculinity, it dominates reporting and soaks up sponsorship to the detriment of other sports, and it pays its stars excessive amounts of money. But even I can see its power to form a bond here, to emphasise common ground. For a moment, I am grateful for football and reminded of how, when it is at its best, sport breaks down barriers and brings people together.

I run while I am in Bethlehem, of course. It is three weeks before the Brighton Marathon and although there is not time to do everything on my training plan, I venture out a few times with Paul Northup, a fellow runner and the new director of Greenbelt. Paul had done a lot of running when he was younger, but having four sons within four years has meant that self-indulgent pursuits such as running have had to take a back seat to more mundane but essential activities, such as earning money and making sure everyone has clean clothes to wear.

Now his boys are older, he is making time to run again and has impressive targets for the times he wants to achieve. We get up early to get our fix before the plans for the day begin.

We run in bright sunshine alongside busy roads, getting lost because Google Maps is not very detailed around here. Running provides a welcome space to mull over what we have seen, and to be authentically ourselves in this place. I had worried that it might not be acceptable for women to run here, but although we do not see any other runners, no one pays much attention to us.

There is far more that could be said about this visit to Palestine. These are snapshots only, the impressions I am taking away with me: of the punitive impact of the Israeli occupation on the lives of ordinary people; of the power of solidarity when people come here to get to know Palestinians and stand with them; of the way that sport can break down barriers and build relationships. On the last night we gather in the bar at the hotel and talk about what we have seen and experienced, and what we might do when we get home.

The people we have met have asked us to go back and tell their stories, to let our friends know what life is like here. We are all aware that we are going back to privileged lives, that however hard we try, we will quickly forget the injustice and restrictions we have seen. We want to honour those we have met by keeping their stories alive. We want to work towards a just peace for both Israelis and Palestinians.

Chris has brought lots of groups of people to Palestine over the years. He acknowledges the challenge of acting on what we have seen and experienced. He says, 'Whatever you do, just do it better. Use it to raise awareness of what is happening here.'

I can see how artists might do that – paint pictures, write poems, make films, tell stories. What do I do? I run. But how can running make a difference here?

* * * * *

I spend far too much time WILFing – that 'What am I Looking For?' clicking on internet links that lead you down a rabbit hole miles away from where you started, with no memory of how you got there or what you were originally looking for. But sometimes it produces gold.

In 2012 the Olympic Games would be in Britain and I wanted to find out if Palestine was competing. I discovered that only one athlete had qualified, for the judo competition, but four others had wildcard entries – two swimmers and two runners. One of the runners, Bahaa al-Farra, was due to compete in the 400m and I found out that he had run ten kilometres of the 2012 Gaza Marathon back in March as part of his training. So Gaza has a marathon? I kept clicking.

The Gaza Marathon was first run in 2011, the brainchild of Gemma Connell, a young Australian woman working for UNRWA, the UN agency for Palestinian refugees. She organised the race in order to raise money for the Summer Games that UNRWA runs each year for children in Gaza, a much-needed chance for them to experience moments of fun and normality in the very challenging environment in which they live.

Gaza is marathon-sized, just 26 miles long; the race started at Beit Hanoun in the north and ran along the coast to Rafah on the Egyptian border. Only nine runners did the whole distance that first year, and Gemma was the only woman to run it. It was won by Nader al-Masri, a Gazan Olympic athlete who competed in the 5k race at Beijing in 2008. But over 1,200 Palestinian children took part in relays along the course, running between 1km and 4km in brightly coloured t-shirts and $1m was raised for the Summer Games. The 2012 race had more competitors and a higher profile. And plans were already in place for a race the following year.

I was hooked. I e-mailed UNRWA and got talking to Chris Rose and Paul Northup. I felt a strong yearning to be a part of the race. I expected it to be an enormous challenge; the 2012 race had taken place in driving winds and rain, and I was still very new to the marathon distance, but I wanted to do it more than anything.

Over the next few months we made plans, and looked for other runners to take part. Paul had been in from the start, and Chris decided to make this his first and only marathon. My brother-in-law Steve Baker was keen to come and he recruited a group of his running friends from Devon. They called themselves the Baggy Breakfast Club after their local headland, Baggy Point, that they ran round most weekends, and their commitment to eating bacon butties afterwards. We started training plans and pestered people for sponsorship. Ahmed, a friend of Chris's from Gaza, also signed up to do the race and was going to show us round his country while we were out there.

We watched the news from Gaza closely. It seemed to be a tense time with conflict between Israelis and Palestinians, and even tighter punitive restrictions on Gaza in response. The infrastructure of the country seemed so fragile, we wondered if the race would actually happen, but news from UNRWA stayed positive and we kept our sights on Gaza.

And then, one month before the race, we got some news that brought an end to those dreams. Hamas, the Islamist governing authority in the Gaza Strip, told UNRWA that the race needed to respect Gaza's local customs; in other words, they would not allow women to compete alongside men. That put UNRWA in an impossible position: host a race for men only which would conflict with their commitment to gender equality, or cancel the race. They chose the latter. Almost half of both the local Palestinian and the international runners who had signed up for the 2013 race were women.

I had expected that as a woman I would have to run with my body more covered up than I would choose, but I was devastated to hear that the race wasn't going to happen at all. The decision by Hamas felt very destructive to me; rather than the marathon being an opportunity to highlight the restrictions and poverty that people have to live with and the need for creative activities for children, Gaza was in the news because their own government was not letting women run.

Chris started to explore alternatives and we frantically swapped e-mails over the course of the day. UNRWA was encouraging people to travel to Gaza anyway and were planning to put on a programme of events and places to visit instead, but we were in the middle of marathon training and wanted to run a race. Fortunately they also let Chris know about a new marathon that was due to take place in Bethlehem about ten days after the Gaza race, the Right to Movement Palestine Marathon being organised by a couple of Danish women, Signe Fischer Smidt and Laerke Hein. We signed up and changed our travel plans.

A few of our group couldn't make the new date, including my brother-in-law Steve, but Chris's friend Ahmed had to drop out for a different reason. Even though he was a Palestinian with a British passport, even though the West Bank and Gaza are technically the same country, as a resident of Gaza he would be extremely unlikely to get permission to travel to the West Bank. The pointless injustice of his exclusion made us even more determined than ever to run a good race and to make it count.

A couple of weeks before we were due to leave for Bethlehem, Chris called us all together to talk about what to expect on the trip. It was great to meet some of the other people who would be running. Bob Mayo is a priest in Shepherd's Bush. He had a speaking engagement the day before the marathon that he did not want to miss and so he would be flying out to Bethlehem overnight, arriving just before the start of the race on the Sunday morning. He was determined to finish the story, to run the race, even though he would be going from tube, to plane, to car, to starting line.

Bob has been running for years, and as he introduced himself to us, he talked about what he particularly loved about it. 'When I run at six in the morning, the streets are mine, the city is mine. Running is a subversive act,' he said. That phrase stuck in my mind and got me thinking.

Running subverts gender stereotypes and cultural traditions, as evidenced in Gaza where the thought of women running alongside men was so abhorrent to Hamas that it was banned. It is only relatively recently that women have been allowed to run long distances; women didn't compete in the Olympic marathon until 1984. Bobbi Gibb ran the Boston Marathon years before that in 1966 after being denied an official place, to the fury of the organisers who very ungraciously conceded that while she had run along the course while the race was happening, she had not run *in* the Boston Marathon. The following year Kathrine Switzer was famously accosted while she was running in the same race by an official who tried to physically drag her to the sidelines.

In these days, when so many women run, I am grateful for these running pioneers who challenged the status quo, subverting the received wisdom that women were too delicate to run more than a few hundred metres, and paved the way for me to do what I love. I loved the fact that it was women who had dreamed into being both the Gaza and the Palestine marathons, having the vision to see what a race could do, and the tenacity to make it happen.

Running subverts the pressure on women to be obsessed with their appearance. There will always be a few women who turn up for races with a full face of make-up but when you run you really don't have to worry about what you look like. I throw on the same kit time after time, often leaving it on the radiator to dry after a short run and putting it on again the following day; I reason that I have worn it for less than an hour and it is not that smelly.

I stuff my unwashed hair in a ponytail or under a hat. I get hot and sweaty and go red in the face, and it doesn't matter at all. I experience my body as strong and capable, rather than something to reduce through diets or put on display. I am amazed at how it works and how well it serves me.

Running subverts the experience of living in a city, helping you reclaim the streets, redeem the commute, seek out the green spaces and river paths, and the parks and trails that are waiting to be found. It is about taking charge of the way you move through urban spaces, owning the routes and choosing how you travel along them. It contradicts the idea that outdoor spaces are not safe for women to be in.

And it subverts the urban interaction with outdoors, which sometimes feels like an inconvenient space between home, tube and workplace. I have done my fair share of moaning about cold winters but I run whatever the weather – in rain, sleet, hail, snow, in the dark, under grey skies, through twilight and especially in sunshine. I have spent hours running outdoors in the cold, dark winter months and it always does my soul good.

Running subverts ideas about competition and achievement. When you start running later in life like I did, it is not about winning races or being the best in a group. It is about exploring what your body can do, how far it can go and trying to go further, how it feels to run a marathon, how to develop the mental endurance that enables you to persevere when you want to give up. It is about being the best you can be and discovering who you are deep down.

So yes, I will always want to better my times, and if there is a person just in front of me near the finishing line I will try to overtake them. But the person I am wanting to beat is myself and that is as much about mental endurance as it is about physical speed.

And of course, in Palestine, where movement is so restricted, where people are separated from their family, land and friends by eight-metre-high concrete barriers, where it is not possible to travel 26.2 miles in a straight line without encountering road blocks, when people from the Gaza Strip are forbidden to exit their tiny besieged enclave and travel to the West Bank, then running a marathon is a wonderfully subversive act.

The Palestine Marathon aimed to highlight just these issues and to promote the right to movement under article 13 of the Universal Declaration of Human Rights: Everyone has the right to freedom of movement and residence within the borders of each state. Everyone has the right to leave any country, including his own, and to return to his country. The invitation to participate said, 'We run to tell a different story than the one of conflict and hate. We want to move. Move with us.'

* * * * *

Race day started at 5am in the hotel lobby. Some people in our team were mixing pots of instant porridge; I was eating pitta bread, hummus and za'atar, a fragrant mix of herbs and spices that is found all over Palestine. The usual advice is 'nothing new on race day' but I wanted the whole authentic Palestinian experience.

We had arrived in Bethlehem a few days before after flying in to Ben Gurion airport in Tel Aviv. We had spent a day walking round Jerusalem as well as another exploring Bethlehem itself, so that everyone could see some of the wider context. Marwan Fararjeh, our guide from the previous year and now our friend, was delighted to see us again, although overtly bemused as to why we were planning to run that far. Marwan is a warm and effusive man, tactile and quick to laugh. Whenever we got out of the minibus, he lit a roll-up cigarette. He waved his arms around as he talked, animated and passionate as he recounted his experiences of living under occupation, determined that we grasp what life is like for him and his family. 'We do run,' he said, 'just usually away from something.'

Our hotel was a short walk away from Manger Square where the race was due to start. We had done a quick recce of the route the day before. Because of the restrictions on travel the race was two laps of an out and back course along the road towards Hebron to the south, with the turnaround at a checkpoint. My heart had sunk when I saw the incline on the out section, a steady rise over miles four to six, then downhill to the turnaround which meant a nasty uphill at the start of the return leg. My hopes of finishing in less than four hours on this course had quietly evaporated at that point, and I felt really apprehensive as I walked to the start.

At home, races run on closed roads will be confirmed as traffic-free before the race is allowed to start, with barriers lining the route at key points to separate runners and spectators. Here in Bethlehem there were cars on the route 30 minutes before the race start time, people rushing to get to where they needed to be, reluctant to submit to yet more restrictions on their travel until they absolutely had to. It was hard to escape the irony that the Right to Movement Marathon was holding up the traffic for a morning.

We gathered in Manger Square under gloomy skies, waiting for the race to start. Usually in April Palestine is all sunshine and warmth, and we had been told to expect temperatures of up to 30 degrees. In fact we seemed to have brought typical British weather with us, drizzle and cold to match the conditions we had trained in. There was a half-marathon and 10k happening at the same time as the marathon, but even so there were fewer than 500 people lined up at the start.

As we waited, my apprehension was overtaken by the palpable sense of excitement in the air. There was lots of chatter, people finding out where each other had come from and what had brought us there. In one sense this was just another race, but it was also so much more than that; it felt like history was being made.

Earlier that same week, explosions at the finish line of the Boston Marathon had killed three people and injured many more. The targeting of terror at a running race had been deeply shocking, one of those moments that makes you recalibrate your perspective of which places are safe and which are risky. The shockwaves had been felt by other sporting events. The London Marathon was taking place on the same day as the Palestine Marathon, and the organisers had done a serious review of their security, deciding eventually that they would go ahead.

The first time I travelled to Palestine, I had had several people ask me how dangerous it was to visit; the bombs in Boston showed that nowhere was immune from terror and in fact Bethlehem felt a very safe place to be. There were two people doing the marathon that day who had also run in Boston, and their presence brought a sense of connection to all those who had suffered so many miles away. There had been a candlelit vigil in Manger Square the night before to honour the victims and we were invited to join a moment of silence before the race began, just as they would do in London later that day.

Bob had turned up in a taxi as the race organisers were doing the briefing through loudspeakers; there was little time to do more than say hello to him and pose for a quick team photo before we gathered on the start line. There was that moment's pause that you get at the start of every race while we stood with fingers hovering over our Garmins, and then we were off.

Most of the marathon runners in our group had planned to set off together and do the first mile at a steady nine-minute pace, but when it came to it we all went our separate ways, caught up in the moment. The race headed out towards the main checkpoint into Bethlehem, and then turned down a side road so that we ran with the wall towering above us on our right.

We ran through Aida Refugee Camp and under the arch that bears a huge key, a tangible expression of people's longing to return to the homes their parents and grandparents had to flee from during the Nakba – the disaster – of the 1948 war. On the walls around the camp are paintings of the villages they had left, place names deliberately listed and honoured so they will not be forgotten. I got quite emotional running past these memorials, aware of how easy it would be for me to visit them while the people who had actually lived there were denied that right.

There were a few spectators on the course, but not many. This was probably the first formal running race that many people had seen, and it was clear that they weren't quite sure what to make of it. I tried to raise some support as I ran, encouraging people to cheer and clap, but quickly gave that up as too exhausting. Palestinian security officers stared at us from their stations, while the police kept impatient drivers in check as we ran past blocked junctions.

But it was the children who made it special. We ran past the UN schools on the edge of Deheishe refugee camp. There was a huge crowd of boys standing outside their school and you could hear their cheers and whistles as you approached up the hill. The girls were harder to spot hanging out of the windows on the top floor of their building, but still waving and shouting in support. Guides and scouts were on duty at the many water stations, handing out fruit, dates and water. And then there were children waving from the windows of their houses, calling out our names which were written in Arabic on our shirts and smiling in delight when we waved back.

I collected a band at the checkpoint to prove I had been there and headed back the way I had come. The uphill section that I had laboured over on the way out was now a welcome downhill but running back into Manger Square I knew that it was time to do it all again.

This second half of the race was hard and lonely. There were only just over 50 people doing the full marathon, and we were really spread out so most of the time I was running on my own. I choose not to listen to music in races, mainly so I can be in the moment, but that does make the moment more painful to be in and I wished I had some upbeat music to keep me going. I had done the first half in just under two hours, and managed to keep running back to the checkpoint, but then walked up the hill after the turnaround.

Once I had walked, it was too easy to lapse into that again, and the second half of my race was much slower. The number of spectators had dwindled further by this second lap. The police were still directing traffic at junctions but with so few runners, cars definitely had priority and I found myself shouting 'runner coming through' several times, and wishing I knew how to say it in Arabic. Still, the guides and scouts were faithfully handing out water, almost competing with each other to be the one to hand it over now the runners were few and far between.

Going into the race, I was pleased with the training I had done. My last six long runs averaged 20 miles each and although I didn't follow my training plan to the letter like I did for Brighton the year before, I had consistently put in the miles. The thing I find most difficult about marathon running is the mental endurance it requires when the going gets tough and this time it was my mind that let me down. I finished in 4 hours 12 minutes.

But actually once I had stopped running and found out how other people had got on, my time felt insignificant compared to the sheer joy of having completed the race. Ali Smith, one of the Devon crew, was third fastest woman overall and we grinned with delight as she was awarded a shield in a ceremony that we didn't understand at all.

Paul was the first international finisher and finished in fourth place. Bob had listened to Handel's *Messiah* as he ran and made a point of getting children to run alongside the route with him. Chris finished in obvious pain, vowing 'never again', but he ran the race without once walking.

I found out later that I had finished in the top ten of an international marathon; I was the seventh fastest woman overall, an achievement that sounds quite impressive until you discover that only eight women completed the race. All of us found it an incredible experience and I came away thinking that it was the happiest race I had ever run.

For years I had experienced running as a route to well-being, something that brought me joy, made me fit, and kept me mentally well. This race in Palestine brought a whole new dimension to my running experience. This was running as a form of protest, as a powerful act of solidarity and as an expression of a human right. We were not just taking part in a race, we were saying that we see what is going on here; we are with you.

Running a marathon is about a commitment to long-term goals, to putting in the hours now in the expectation that it will bear fruit in the future. I was inspired by the sense of defiant hope that I saw among many of the Palestinians I met, and their commitment to building a better future even though the present seems to get more difficult year on year. There will be no quick fix; it needs tenacity and commitment. Marwan said to us, 'I know that the first hundred years of my struggle will be hard,' and in some small way running the marathon helped me understand that better.

We went out to run a race and we came back humbled to have met some great people, with our eyes opened to what is happening in the land called Holy. It is hard to say whether we had changed anything by being there, but I know that running the first Palestine Marathon had changed us.

* * * * *

So we made plans to go back in 2014. Bob was keen to run it again, as was Ali. My sister-in-law Susie Baker signed up to do her first half-marathon, and was joined by her friends Tracey Elliott and Jaqs Waggett whose partners had done it the year before; there seemed to be a growing affinity between their Devon village and Bethlehem. Chris was contacted by a guy called Asad from Birmingham who had heard that Amos was leading a trip and wanted to come along; we welcomed him on to the team.

Knowing from experience what the course was like, I tried to include more hills in my training, making more frequent trips to Richmond Park for my long runs. I still did most of my long runs solo because I knew that I would likely be running on my own in Bethlehem again, but also because most people avoid hills on their long runs rather than seeking them out like me.

Getting into Israel was more eventful this time. Asad, a British Pakistani Muslim, got held up at passport control at Ben Gurion airport. I stayed with him in a dull waiting room with various other travellers who had been deemed suspicious for one reason or another, while Chris took the rest of the group on to the hotel. We were both questioned a number of times by a bored but unwavering security guard. Eventually, after six hours, we were let through and got a taxi to Bethlehem, joining the rest of our team at the hotel for a late supper.

The following evening, we discovered that Ali was also having a difficult time getting into the country. She had been on holiday with her family in the States, and so was joining us the night before the race, travelling on her own from Heathrow. The Israeli airline she was travelling with subjected her to some quite unpleasant questioning and searches because she was a woman travelling on her own, and she thought at one point she would not be allowed on the flight. I went back to Ben Gurion to meet her, quietly fuming that people on our team were being so inconvenienced.

At the same time I was highly aware that it was all part of the reason we were there, to highlight the restrictions that so many Palestinian people face as they try to travel and to call for the right to movement for everyone. It made for a late night before the marathon, but it also fuelled my sense of injustice and made me determined to run a good race.

The race had more than doubled in size across all distances for its second edition with 150 people starting the marathon, 350 doing the half and over 600 doing the 10k. Running clubs had been set up in the local towns of Beit Sahour and Ramallah during the year, and they had clearly got people ready for the race. In the UK every town worth its salt has some kind of race, whether that is a 10k, half-marathon or marathon. This race said that Bethlehem was a town just like any other, while at the same time bringing something extra special to it.

This year the weather was hot and sunny rather than cold and wet, which made for a harder race although it felt more authentically Middle Eastern. This time round I paced my run better, and all the hills I had done in training paid off. I still didn't manage to run all the way, but I conquered the four-hour barrier and finished in 3:58.05. When I found out three months later that this time had got me a Good for Age place in the London Marathon in 2015 because by then I would be 50, I cried genuine tears of joy. It felt very fitting that the race which had won my heart should be the place where I got my first sub-four PB.

* * * * *

By the time I returned to Palestine in April 2015, I had damaged my knee with that fall in Richmond Park and I had also found a lump in my right breast. I had an appointment at my GP lined up for my return, and didn't tell anyone else about it, apart from Jonny. I managed to put my anxiety to one side while I was in Bethlehem. This time my sister Mandy came to do the half, and Paul was back to give the marathon another go. At one point I had thought I might not be able to run, but after a few appointments with a physio, my knee was recovered enough for me to attempt the 10k. It would have felt strange to have been there and not run at all.

The race had grown in numbers again and this year even Marwan was going to run the 10k. The marathon and half started first, so I waved off the rest of the team and waited for my turn to race with Marwan and his son Mohammed. Just before the race started they had released doves, and balloons in the colours of the Palestinian flag. Marwan was close to tears as he talked about the pride he felt in the race being staged in his town, about the increased confidence he saw in his people and the hope it gave him. 'One day, like those doves, we'll be free,' he said.

The marathon and half had attracted a lot of international competitors, but the runners in the 10k were mainly local Palestinians and it had a real festival atmosphere. The race was a mix of speedy runners and those who intended to walk it right from the start. I set off with Marwan and his son, but after a while pulled ahead because I wanted to get back before the other Amos runners finished their half-marathon.

I ran slowly drinking in the atmosphere, stopping to take photos as I went, cheering people on and high-fiving children on the way. I felt a twinge of sadness at having to turn round at the 10k point instead of carrying on down the half-marathon route towards Hebron, but the pain in my knee told me that I had made the right decision not to do any more than the shortest distance.

The plus side of doing the 10k was that I was there in Manger Square to take photos of our team as they finished, and encourage them up the final incline to the finish line. And I saw Nader al-Masri, the Gazan athlete, win the marathon after two years of not being allowed to travel to take part in the race, a really emotional moment.

So I didn't get to do what I had wanted in Palestine that year, but the alternative I discovered was great. I headed back home to find out what the doctor had to say.

4

Diagnosis
April and May

HERE is a fact that I will have to live with for the rest of my life. At some point I noticed that the shape of my chest at the top of my breast was different on my right side to my left. I can't tell you exactly when I first saw it because I chose to ignore it. Every so often I would stand in front of the mirror after a shower and turn from side to side to see whether the difference was still there, and it was. I will never know how much easier this last year would have been if I had done something about it as soon as I noticed it.

But it was a while before I acknowledged the anxiety humming quietly at the edge of my consciousness. And then I just knew that I mustn't ignore it any longer. I felt both my breasts and found an unmistakeable lump in the right one, and wondered why on earth I had not done that before.

A lump can mean a number of things. But of course my mind shrieked 'cancer!' at me even while I tried to reassure myself. I rang my doctor's surgery and asked for an urgent appointment, only to find that it wasn't urgent in their eyes so I arranged to see someone in three weeks' time when I came back from Palestine.

I am hardly ever ill and had rarely visited the surgery. When the appointment came round, it was with a male doctor I had never seen before. He felt the lump, while a chaperone hovered in the corner, and told me it was nothing to worry about; there were no extra indications to suggest it was cancerous but he would send me for a hospital check-up just to make sure. How quickly we take our cues from the experts who know more than us. I chided myself for being anxious and got on with life.

Two weeks later I went by myself to Ealing Hospital for a mammogram, expecting it to be nothing more than a quick examination with the results to come later. My breasts were stretched by the technician and squashed by the machine while I stood in ungainly positions trying to hold my arms out of the way. I was sent to have an ultrasound on my right breast, and lay there trying to interpret the comments and facial expressions of the sonographer. Was this anything unusual? Was she concerned by what she was looking at?

Next came a wait outside the consultant's office in an ugly, cramped waiting room. I felt uneasy and out of place. Did I have anything in common with the other women waiting here? Was this somewhere that would become familiar?

My name was called. Ms Shah, the consultant, introduced herself and the breast cancer nurse accompanying her. For the third time that morning I took off my top and bra, this time so that she could examine me for herself. Then clothed, and sitting across the desk from her, came my moment of truth.

'Do you want to know what I think?'

'Yes.'

'I think it is cancer.'

'Why?'

'This is my job. I see this all the time.'

She sent me down to the ultrasound room again, to have a biopsy taken of the lump and some cells taken from a swollen lymph node under my arm. Waiting to be seen, I started to write myself a training plan for the North Devon Marathon at the end of June. My knee had finally recovered after my pre-Palestine fall in Richmond Park and I wanted to get back into condition for the ultra that I was planning to do that autumn. I had not run much for a couple of months but I hoped that it wouldn't take too long to get my fitness back. One part of my brain was telling me how ridiculous this was, that I was unlikely to be running a marathon anytime soon.

Another part was defiantly in denial, and working out how many long runs I could fit in over the next ten weeks. The words 'I think it is cancer' hung in a cartoon speech bubble in my head; I had heard them, but I wasn't allowing them to land anywhere that could feel them or analyse them.

It was the same sonographer. Top and bra off again. Back on the couch with my arm above my head. Prodding and pushing to find the lumps and snatch bits from them. Clothes back on. Home.

A 'might be' diagnosis is a strange thing. It opens the door to the worst possibilities without any facts to ground them or any way to discern which to pay attention to. I had ten days to get through before my next appointment with Ms Shah to find out for sure. I rang Jonny when I got back home and told him that I might have cancer. A phone call at work was perhaps not the easiest way for him to get the news but I wanted him to know what I knew as soon as possible.

We had met at university when we were both doing maths degrees and had got married the summer that we graduated. We had had our two boys soon afterwards. Knowing how easy it was for men and women to slot into narrow, stereotypical roles without even thinking about it, we had always been intentional about sharing equally the hands-on parenting and domestic work that accompanies small children, so that all of us had the opportunity to thrive. We had job-shared a role in a youth work charity when Joel and Harry were small, we each worked part-time when they first went to school and then worked full-time again as they got older and more independent. Our life together had been a busy but fulfilling jumble of juggling responsibilities and trying not to drop anything.

Like most families, there were periods of tag-team parenting where it felt like we hardly saw each other, but those were interlaced with enough time together to keep reminding us why we had said 'I do' all those years before. Jonny had always encouraged me to learn and grow and had held space open for me in which I could flourish. He had shown me how to chill out and to take myself less seriously. I hated having to tell him I had cancer because I knew that it would cause him pain, but I also knew that he would be with me in whatever was to happen next and I didn't want to do it without him.

We also told Joel, his wife Kat, and Harry what was happening a few days later because they were all staying at our house for the weekend and Harry was about to go into his degree finals. I wanted to give him as much time as I could to adjust to the news before he had to sit his exams. It is a horrible thing to have to tell your children you have cancer. They were young adults living away from home so they were not dependent on us like they had been when they were small.

Joel was running his own business as a graphic designer. He had met Kat at school and they had got married the year before, a sparkling day in the story of our family that still made me smile every time I thought about it. Just after Christmas they had told us that they were expecting a baby, casually dropping this momentous news into a conversation about camping. Harry was somehow juggling his maths and German degree with his burgeoning career as a spoken word artist, taking every opportunity that came his way to travel and perform even if that meant missing lectures, and teaching himself his maths modules in bouts of frenzied revision just before assignments and exams.

So I was at the stage of life where the word 'mother' had shifted from being a verb, something that I actively did to nurture my children, to being a noun, a description of the relationship that still bound us together even though they needed me far less these days. But still as a parent, you want to be strong, to be there for your children, not to cause them anxiety and pain. We had had breakfast together around the kitchen table and Harry was about to head off somewhere when I said, 'I need to tell you something,' and broke the news. Harry, who wears his heart on his sleeve, dissolved into tears. Joel, who processes everything internally, looked dismayed and I was so glad that Kat was there to support him. As a paediatric oncology nurse she, perhaps more than all of us, knew what the next few months would hold.

But I told very few other people in those days of maybe having cancer. I wanted to be able to give my family and friends details of exactly what was wrong and what would happen next, rather than plunging them into the same distortion of reality that I was experiencing. I realised that imagining the worst would not make it any more or less likely to happen, and I tried to stay with what I knew rather than start planning my funeral service.

But it was hard to concentrate at work with the word 'cancer' throbbing through my head, or to be fully engaged with anything. I felt distracted, and distant from the people who did not know what was occupying my thoughts. My early morning runs over the next few days were a cathartic and welcome space where I could just be myself. Anxiety and fear swirled around my mind for the first couple of miles as I allowed myself to face the reality of what was happening but then settled into the background, calmed into perspective by the meditative rhythm of my feet on the ground and the space to just be. I arrived home each time thinking, 'Whatever happens, you can do this.'

In fact, just a week later I was back at the hospital with Jonny, having been called back early because of a mix-up over appointment times. We found out that Ms Shah's initial thoughts were right; it was breast cancer and it was in at least one of my lymph nodes. I was expecting to have the diagnosis confirmed after what she had said the week before, but it was still hard to hear and difficult to take in. Over the next couple of weeks I had MRI and CT scans to see if the cancer had spread. Those scans revealed a shadow on my liver and fibroids in my womb, so I had more ultrasound tests to investigate those further. I had to go for another biopsy of a gristly lump they found in the same breast;

it took several attempts by the sonographer to get enough tissue, leaving me bruised and sore.

It was remarkable to discover just how many lumps and bumps my body was host to. Each time a new one was identified the fear would rise again that it was something serious, an added complication to what we already knew. It was a weird fortnight because this was all happening behind the scenes of my normal life. Some days I would go to work and then leave at lunchtime, ostensibly to work from home for the afternoon, but really for a hospital appointment. I had not been to hospital for years; now I seemed to be there every few days. Fortunately the other lumps and bumps were discounted as nothing to worry about; it was only the ones in my breast and armpit that were a cause for concern.

Does anyone expect to get cancer? I certainly did not and having the diagnosis confirmed was a shock. I had been sent a routine mammogram appointment for later in the year because I was turning 50, and I knew that the risk of getting cancer grew with age but I was fit, I had only smoked the odd cigarette here and there, I exercised regularly, ate healthily; all these things that we trust to make us invincible had failed me. I was floundering around trying to make sense of it.

Someone on the medical team told us not to read about cancer on the internet, which is impossible advice in this digital age; we go online to find a recipe for lemon curd, to discover which other films that actor starred in, to find out how much houses are selling for down our road. Of course, I was going to look online to find out as much information as I could about what was happening to me; it would have been more constructive if they had told me which sites would give me accurate information.

It takes a moment to get a diagnosis; it takes longer to realise the full implications. Up until now, CANCER was an upper-case catastrophe that happened to other people. Now it was an unwelcome part of my world and I was discovering just how multi-faceted and diverse it was. I read up about grades and stages of cancer, inducting myself into a new language of diagnoses and treatments, acronyms and abbreviations, finding out that breast cancer is one of the more treatable, but that 30 women in the UK still die from it every day. The story of cancer that I was familiar with was of a person getting steadily more ill but not knowing why, until their doctor does tests and announces the bad news. That was not my story. I couldn't get over how well I felt and how that seemed so inconsistent with a cancer diagnosis. How could I have cancer when I could cycle 50 miles at the weekend and run to work during the week? I soaked up information but I was still none the wiser about exactly what it meant for me.

So I took charge of what I could, which was letting other people know about it. While I was waiting to find out the diagnosis I had made lists of who to tell and when to tell them as a way of holding on to some kind of control when it felt like everything was shifting. I rang my three sisters and arranged to see my mum, Mary Slark, telling her that my sister Mandy and I were going to take her out for a belated Mothers' Day lunch. My dad had died about 18 months before and although my mum was adapting to her new single life brilliantly I wanted to tell her what was going on face to face.

I am the second oldest in the family and Mandy is two years younger than me. We didn't get on that well as small children; I felt she was my dad's favourite and was rather jealous of her, but I had got to know her again as an adult when she had moved to London to train as a pub manager and we had become really close. She is quite different to me: her hair is auburn where mine is dark brown; she is an extrovert who can talk easily to anyone whereas I am an introvert who takes time to get to know people; she is a skilled craftswoman who runs her own business while I do most of my work on a computer.

But she is my go-to fashion adviser whenever I need to buy new clothes and I know she would do anything for me. She lives in Essex and I got the tube to the end of the Central Line where she picked me up and drove me to our mum's house in Ely. We talked and cried in the car on the way, a helpful dress rehearsal for what I would say to my mum a couple of hours later. We did take my mum out for lunch, but only after I told her in her kitchen, over cups of coffee and almond macaroons, that I had breast cancer. Telling my family brought tears each time, but also a strong sense of being held in their love and the knowledge that they would be there for me; I was not going to have to do this alone.

Telling other people was harder. I could be real about how I was feeling with close friends, but it wasn't appropriate to be completely vulnerable with everyone when I was still coming to terms with it myself. Sometimes I found myself having to manage other people's shock and grief, reassuring them that it would be all right when I was far from certain about that myself.

Sometimes my news came on top of other stresses in people's lives that I didn't know about. One of my work colleagues dissolved into tears when I told her, but that was as much about the other stuff she was having to deal with as it was how she felt about me. I found that I could influence people's reactions by the way I told them, but that I needed to be in a good place in myself before I broke the news. I didn't want people's pity and I think that sometimes meant I was tougher than I needed to be. I felt that I needed to direct the cast of family, friends, work colleagues and onlookers, to set the tone of how I wanted this to go, so that no one else would take the reins. I was grasping for shreds of control because I felt that I had so little.

But there is no action plan that is handed to you along with your diagnosis, telling you how to do cancer. You make it up as you go along.

Mandy and I went to watch the London Marathon along with lots of Eagles from my running club. Harry had a charity place from Amos Trust and was raising money for their work in Palestine. I had written him a training plan a few months previously but studies, poetry gigs, the social demands of student life and the confidence of youth meant he largely ignored it. Harry throws himself wholeheartedly into life, turning every opportunity into an adventure, and a couple of weeks before the race he decided that he wanted to run with a representation of the Bethlehem separation wall on his back.

I told him he was mad. It was going to be hard enough running a marathon on the little training he had done let alone with a heavy, wind-resistant barrier on his back. He ignored that too, constructing a two-metre-high 'wall' out of a backpack, bamboo canes and gaffer tape. He had run across London with it the week before the marathon, to try it out, having at least listened to my 'nothing new on race day' advice and also to get it to Greenwich where Joel and Kat very conveniently lived a few roads away from the start of the race. His wall made him very easy to spot in the crowds, and we had no trouble cheering him on near mile six and then at mile 23 where the Eagles have a huge presence. It did my heart good to see his determination and compassion for other people.

Watching the marathon, it was hard to escape just how many people were running for cancer charities. There was a large group of Macmillan supporters just opposite where we were standing at mile six, and it seemed that everywhere I looked there were runners with Breast Cancer Care, or Marie Curie, or Bloodwise or Cancer Research logos on their shirts. It is probably similar to the phenomenon of seeing pregnant women everywhere once you decide you want a baby; cancer was at the top of my mind and it was not surprising that I saw it all around me. I teared up thinking about the reasons why those people were running for those charities, for their mums, their children, their friends, a story of pain and hope motivating each of them.

Another hospital appointment brought the beginning of a treatment plan. I needed chemotherapy first to try and shrink the tumour, then a full mastectomy because there was a second smaller tumour in the breast as well as the large one I had found, and probably radiotherapy and hormone therapy to finish. I was given a date to see the oncologist who would decide exactly what chemotherapy I needed. It would be exactly a month since that first meeting with Ms Shah; it felt much longer.

The enormity of what was happening was starting to sink in. I felt like cancer was pushing me into a parallel reality to everyone else where I could observe what they were doing but couldn't join in. My world was dramatically changing while everyone else was carrying on as normal. I felt like an exhibit, with people watching me to see how I was coping. I felt fragile, diminished, and isolated. My very identity was being challenged; if I was not the fit, busy, efficient one, then who was I? I oscillated between thinking on my better days that this was no big deal, to thinking that I was losing my life as I knew it. The familiar structure of work, running, and social life was disappearing and I didn't know how to negotiate the space that had opened up in its place

And I found I had really conflicting feelings about my body. On the one hand, I had got to a stage in my life where I really appreciated my body and felt very at home in my skin. Women are conditioned from such an early age to criticise their bodies and to invest time, energy and money in trying to perfect them. We are told that we are too fat, too hairy, too wrinkly, and too smelly, and so we diet, we wax, we smooth, and we deodorise. We cover up our blemishes and dye our grey hair. We suck in our stomachs and squeeze our feet into high-heeled shoes that cause us pain and stop us being able to move freely. I was no more immune to this onslaught than anyone else but I had learned to challenge internally those feelings of being physically inadequate when they arose, and was starting to be pissed off with them.

I had got over the awkward clumsiness I had experienced as a teenager when my feet and limbs grew so fast they seemed hard to control. I had grown out of wishing I was small and delicate and had learned to stand tall, even though I towered over most of my friends. I was proud of the physical things my body had enabled me to do. This body had nurtured and given birth to my two amazing sons, and I had grown to accept the slightly squidgy mummy tummy they had left me with. This body had helped me to achieve some tough physical challenges. It had carried me through five marathons and numerous triathlons. It had shown me I could do things that I thought were beyond me. Why should I be made to feel that my body was not good enough?

But at the same time I felt betrayed by the body that I had grown to love. This cancer was not an alien thing that had invaded my breast from outside; it was my own cells that had dangerously mutated and, if left to their own devices, would kill me. While I had been running around Bethlehem, while I had been cycling to work, while I had been digging my allotment those dysfunctional cells were multiplying secretly inside me, creating tumours that would need to be cut out of me. How far had they infiltrated through my body? How much damage had they done already? How much more would they do?

I cried in secret and ranted to Jonny: I don't want to have cancer. I don't want to be ill. I don't want to lose my hair. I don't want to be weak and diminished. I don't want my life to change. I don't want to lose my breast. I don't want to be left out of all the things I had planned to do this year. I don't want to be brave and stoical. I don't want to be pitied. I don't want this.

But this was happening in spite of my ranting, and my plans for the year were dissolving in front of me. I didn't know what this diagnosis would mean for my running and so far I had been running at every opportunity, a sense of urgency driving me to make the most of it while I still could. My knee had fully recovered by now after the fall in Richmond Park and I was back to doing ten miles at the weekends. But there was no escaping the fact that this return to fitness was not going to lead to what I had hoped.

The North Devon Marathon had always been a bit of a pipe dream and I had to concede it was impossible for me to do it this year. I had to let go of the Bath Two Tunnels Marathon and the 50k race I had planned for the autumn. I was on the women's Welsh Castles Relay team for the Eagles at the beginning of June, a prestigious 20-stage race over two days from Caernarfon to Cardiff. I e-mailed Jen Watt, the team captain, to let her know that I wouldn't be able to do it so she could get one of the reserves to step up instead.

The one event that I was holding on to with grim determination was a cycle ride to Amsterdam with Amos Trust that was in the diary for the end of May. I had no idea whether I would be able to do it, but I chose to assume that I could and to keep training for it anyway. With so much of what I had planned for the year being taken away from me, it was tempting to just give up on everything but I decided that I was not going to let go of this one until I knew that it was going to be taken from me.

Jonny and I went to see the oncologist, Dr Lewanski, an upbeat man who managed to stay cheerful even while reciting all the worst side-effects of chemotherapy. It is so easy to become passive as a patient, to trust specialists without thinking because they are the experts who know what they are talking about. You are advised to think through in advance the questions you want to ask your doctors, and to take a list. As well as wanting to understand what was happening to me and the treatment that was being proposed, I had one main concern. Would I be able to run over the next few months? And could I run to my chemotherapy sessions?

Dr Lewanski was intrigued; no one had ever asked him that before but he didn't see why not. It turned out that he was a marathon runner and we swapped stories of races in between talking about the constipation, nausea and hair loss that were heading my way. He sang the praises of German marathons because of their efficient organisation and suggested I should try Berlin next. I left hopeful that although I was losing so many things, perhaps I would not completely lose my running.

When you get a cancer diagnosis you are assigned to a multi-disciplinary medical team with specialists for each of the different types of treatment you will need. They write to each other about their proposals for treatment and as the patient you get a copy, a process that feels quaintly old-fashioned but which allows you to eavesdrop on their conversation and have a copy in writing of what they discussed with you in person at your appointment. In the letter that Dr Lewanksi wrote to Ms Shah, he described me as a runner and included my marathon PB. I felt really touched, as if he had seen who I really was and was acknowledging what was most important to me. He was a golden moment in a dark and difficult time.

And something shifted for me after that appointment. The year before, in 2014, after my sub-four marathon in Palestine,

I had signed up for the Chester Marathon in the autumn. My goal was to go sub-3:50; I wanted to be able to say that I had got a good-for-age time in my 40s. It was a challenging target, and I tried a new training plan – the lowest mileage one in Pfitzinger and Douglas's *Advanced Marathoning* book. The word 'Advanced' in the title appealed to my vanity, but the book also spelt out a different structure to training and prescribed higher mileage than I had done before. The plan I followed was an 18-week one which had four cycles – increasing your mileage to build endurance, improving your lactate threshold by varying the intensity of your training, preparing for the race by running at your race pace and doing some practice races, and tapering so that you start your marathon on rested legs.

There were hard weeks when you built your mileage and pushed yourself in speed work, and then easier weeks when you let your body acclimatise to the training you had done so far. In the end, I twisted my ankle three weeks before the race so lost momentum and came in at 3:50.14, so I didn't quite hit my target. But the 18-week plan had served me well.

At my appointment, Dr Lewanksi gave me an 18-week plan for chemotherapy. There would be six cycles three weeks apart, with hard weeks just after treatment and hopefully an easier week before the next one. The pattern of it felt strangely familiar, although it would have the opposite effect on my body to that P&D plan. At last I could put dates in my diary of when the promised treatments would be happening, and start to plan around them.

I had had so much information to take in. I had the prospect of surgery in the autumn and then probably radiotherapy and hormone therapy after that. It was hard to get my head round it all, and when I did think about those future stages of treatment, I found myself getting really anxious. Maybe all I needed to do was focus on the next step that was ahead of me. And I knew I could do an 18-week plan.

I had ranted and raged at all that I didn't want to accept about this next stage of my life, but now I started to think more about what I did want, and what I could do to approach it constructively. I had blogged on and off for a while, setting up my blog so I could write about the first Palestine Marathon three years earlier. I had always found solace in writing; the process of crafting words on a page usually helped me to work out what I was thinking and stopped me getting stuck, so I blogged about what was happening to me and linked to it from Facebook.

Everyone has to decide for themselves how they will go through cancer treatment, and how they will interact with the people around them. Not everyone chooses to go public and I understand that. But for me, blogging about my diagnosis was a revelation. There was an outpouring of love and support on Facebook, and it set off a small avalanche of cards, e-mails, letters, flowers and gifts that started arriving at my house over the next few days and that carried on throughout my treatment.

Friends who had had breast cancer or who had supported others through it offered wisdom and practical advice. People got in touch to say they didn't know what to say, but saying that was more than enough. I heard from people that I had not seen for years, as well as those that were part of my everyday life. I felt loved, and seen, and held.

And some people said just what I needed to hear. Since the diagnosis, I had struggled to pray, unsure of what to say or how God fitted into what was happening, even though I have had a faith since childhood. Maggi Dawn, a friend who is a theology professor in the States, sent these words to me, 'Once upon a time, I went on a retreat in a monastery. I was excessively tired, and not very well. I remember thinking to myself, "Why did I come on retreat? Now I will have to pray, and I really can't be bothered." The monk who met me at the door and showed me to my room told me all about the routine, the meals, the chapel services etc. And then he said, "By the way, don't feel you have to pray all day long. I sense that you are here because you need others to pray for you. We are praying for you, so you should just rest." Maybe with your friends praying for you all around, you can just rest too, when you don't feel like praying?'

Somehow that gave me permission to just be and to deal with this how I needed to, rather than thinking that there was an ideal response that I ought to have.

That doesn't mean that interactions with other people were always easy or welcome. A few people who I had expected to be supportive withdrew, unable to cope for some reason, which was hurtful at the time. But I had to just let that go; I didn't have the emotional energy to pursue what was going on for them and I wasn't responsible for their reaction. I was still struggling to come to terms with it all, to find any stability in this life that had been knocked off course and, in truth, it was almost impossible at times for people to get it right.

Sometimes everyone irritated me. If someone offered advice or made a suggestion, I would get annoyed that they were interfering. If people said nothing, I would feel isolated and alone. I realised how contrary I was being and also recognised the invitation there was in this to let people love me. I tried to remember that every text, every e-mail, every suggestion, however clumsy, or unwelcome, or mistimed, or appropriate, or helpful or insightful was someone's way of saying I love you and I care about you.

I had to decide what to do about work. I was working for a charity which supported social action by churches and I was in charge of a network of partnerships across England. I travelled regularly for work, to places as far apart as Truro, Manchester and Norwich, and managed a small team of people. I heard really contrasting stories of how chemotherapy affected people. Lots of people talked about extreme fatigue and nausea but then there were also the mythical women who kept working all the way through their treatment so that their colleagues didn't even know they were having it. Who knew how I would respond? How do you plan for something that is so mysterious and unpredictable?

I was acutely aware of how what was happening to me was also happening to my colleagues and would have a huge impact on their workload. I was fortunate that my workplace was very supportive and would continue to pay me for up to six months of sick leave. And so I decided to work one week in every three towards the end of each chemo cycle. I was advised not to travel over the next four months because of the risk of infection so I arranged for other people to visit the partnerships I managed and contacted them to let them know what was happening. With a spreadsheet in place of when I would be in the office, and who was doing what when I was on sick leave, I felt better that at least there was a plan, even if it would all have to be changed once I found out how my body would respond to chemotherapy.

One early conversation I had had with someone in my running club had stayed with me. His partner had chosen not to have chemotherapy when she had breast cancer and she had stayed healthy by changing her diet. I didn't want to go down that same path. My instinct was to trust my doctors and to embrace the treatment they were recommending, but I wanted to find out about the lifestyle choices that would complement mainstream medicine. The official NHS advice is to 'eat a healthy diet' but of course there are many different ways to interpret that. And while the internet is full of controversial cancer diet advice, there is also some good evidence-based research.

I discovered Professor Jane Plant, a geochemist who had investigated environmental causes of cancer and who had had breast cancer six times herself. Intrigued by the fact that women in China and Japan have very low incidences of breast cancer until they move to the West and adopt a Western lifestyle, she researched the impact of diet on cancer. She advocated a vegan diet for people with active cancer and had followed that herself. It made a lot of sense to me and so overnight I cut out meat, fish, eggs and dairy, I filled my fridge with vegetables and my kitchen cupboards with nuts and seeds.

I had read *Eat and Run* by Scott Jurek so I knew that a vegan diet was suitable for a world-class athlete, let alone a runner like me. It was not that I expected this change in diet to cure me of cancer or replace any of the treatment, but it did help me feel that I was giving my body the best chance of coping with the chemotherapy that was to come. I was aware that it could be a bid for control when I had so little control over what was happening to me, but it gave me a sense of agency and it felt like a positive choice towards health.

Having a plan for treatment, choosing to change my diet, sorting out work and starting to write about what was happening to me all helped to restore my equilibrium and gave me back a sense of clarity and purpose. I knew what the next few months would hold and what was required of me. And one of the best things about the chemo plan was that it would allow me to do the Amsterdam cycle ride after all. I would need to come back a day early in order to have blood tests before my first treatment, but I could do it.

For the last few years I had spent the late May Bank Holiday weekend on a cycle ride with people from Amos Trust. The rides had started as a fundraising event for the Street Child World Cup which Amos had initiated several years before, but they had turned into an opportunity for an assorted mix of supporters and friends to cycle and have a laugh together. Over the previous few years we had cycled around the Caledonian Canal in Scotland, had done London to Paris, had cycled the Way of the Roses, the coast-to-coast route across Lancashire and Yorkshire, and had cycled through Flanders to Bruges. This year 18 of us set off on a Saturday morning from St Clements in London, where Amos has its office base, to cycle to Harwich, picking up people at Chelmsford and Colchester en route; others were cycling from Cambridge or driving for the first day, with around 50 people in total cycling over the weekend.

The route out of London was a bit tricky, not helped by a shower of rain. We seemed to go round the Olympic Park a couple of times before working out which way to leave it. But once we were on the NCN route, it was a great ride down country lanes with some sunshine. We stopped in Chelmsford where our van driver had made friends with some builders who made us a cup of tea and let us use their very smelly portaloo. Some confusion about the route near Maldon meant we did a few more miles than we needed to, and by the time we got to Colchester it was getting pretty late.

A few people had gone on ahead, some more piled into the van with their bikes and that left five of us to ride hard to Ramsey where supper and all the other cyclists were waiting for us before the final push to the ferry. There is nothing like that sense of slight desperation about whether you are going to make it in time to help you find energy when you feel like you have got none left. We arrived at the pub to be greeted by the landlord at the door saying, 'Are you Jenny? Your stir-fry is ready.' I could have kissed him.

While I was eating, a text arrived from Lucy Rigg, a fellow runner who was at the Eagles' summer party back in Ealing, to say that I had won my age category in the club championships. With all that was going on, that felt like a pleasing affirmation of what a great year of running I had had over the previous 12 months. It also felt like a full stop and the start of a new paragraph. My running over the next year would be in a very different category.

After a night on the ferry, we set off for Amsterdam. The Dutch have a brilliant system for marking cycle routes. Knooppunten are numbered nodes around the country, and to follow a route you just need to know which order of nodes to travel through. Signs on the route point you towards the next node you are aiming for. It is not infallible and we had to resort to iPhones occasionally, but it is a very flexible and easy system that largely takes you down dedicated cycle routes or quiet roads through beautiful countryside. We cycled through Leiden which seemed to be an idyllic town where everyone had a boat for Sunday afternoon cruising along the canals and we stayed the night in a hostel in Vondelpark in Amsterdam.

On Monday morning, Jonny and I set off to cycle back to the Hook of Holland for the two o'clock ferry while everyone else enjoyed a day in the city. We left at seven in the morning, and went a different route down the coast which was easier to follow. We made it in time, arrived back in England around 8pm, got the train to Stratford, and then had to cycle to Aldgate East to get a tube home because of engineering works.

It was a stark reminder of just how pitiful London's approach to cycling is; instead of the separated routes and respect for cyclists that are so prevalent in Holland, we have a bit of blue paint on the road and aggression from drivers. Still, it was a wonderful weekend and I was so grateful that I was able to do something so physical and so vital. I was secretly pleased that I was the only woman who had cycled all the way to Harwich on that first day and so was the woman who had cycled the furthest over the weekend; having cancer had not quashed my competitive spirit. And cycling over 200 miles seemed an appropriate thing to have done just before chemotherapy, a defiant celebration of the strength of my body, of its capacity to endure, before everything was about to change.

Not What I Had Planned

I was 50 in March and I had lots of running planned this year to celebrate – marathons in Palestine and London, and a 50k coastal race in the autumn with the Bath Two Tunnels Marathon as preparation. Instead I tripped during my last long run before Palestine and ended up with a fantastic black eye and a badly bruised knee which ruled me out of the first two races. And now I have been diagnosed with breast cancer and I am heading into six rounds of chemo with surgery in the autumn.

I can't claim to have any profound or original thoughts but this is where I am with it at the moment.

Life goes on. The day after I found out I had cancer, I went to the theatre with my friend Letty for a belated birthday treat. I told her over supper and cried, but then we had a wonderful evening together, with fab food, conversation and the discovery of Hampstead Theatre. I feel like cancer will dominate my life for a while but I don't want to be defined by it or reduced to it – it is not the only thing that is going on in my life, or in the lives of those I love.

I have set myself lots of physical challenges over the last few years – triathlons, marathons, coast-to-coast cycle rides, the Dunwich Dynamo – and my body has carried me through them all. I have loved going beyond what I thought I could do, and discovering what I am physically and mentally capable of. This is a new physical challenge and not one I would ever have chosen. And it is not going to be some great fitness adventure – it is going to be shit. But I hope my body, mind and spirit will serve me well and carry me through.

RUN FOR YOUR LIFE

I was among the many people who defaced the ridiculous Protein World ads on the tube. They ask, 'Are you beach body ready?' and just after my diagnosis I scrawled on one, 'Honey, this strong body is ready for anything life throws at me.' Actually, I don't know that I am ready for this – how can you be? – but being physically fit and being surrounded by my amazing family and friends will stand me in good stead. And it underlines for me how the message of those adverts is so pernicious; what my body looks like over the next few months is going to be the least significant thing about it.

Instead of running the marathon in Palestine, I ran the 10k and it was delightful. Most of the runners are local people and for many of them, it is their first race. There is such a celebratory and bold feeling to it. I started the race with Marwan and his son and took photos as I ran. I was there when the rest of my group finished their races to cheer them home and take more photos of them finishing. I didn't get to do what I wanted, but the alternative was great. I hope that over the next few months I will discover the delights of things I would have missed if my original plans had worked out.

A Poem For This Year

My friend Grace Wroe gave me a copy of this poem by Rumi for my 50th birthday this year. It stood out at the time among the other birthday wishes for flourishing and good times because it acknowledged a darker possibility which has been very prescient.

The Guesthouse

This being human is a guesthouse.
Every morning a new arrival.

A joy, a depression, a meanness
some momentary awareness comes as an
unexpected visitor.

Welcome and entertain them all!
Even if they are a crowd of sorrows,
who violently sweep your house empty of its
furniture.
Still, treat each guest honourably.
He may be clearing you out for some new delight.

The dark thoughts, the shame, the malice
meet them at the door laughing and invite them in.

Be grateful for whoever comes,
because each has been sent as a guide from
beyond.

I have thought about it a lot. I can identify with that feeling of my house being swept empty, of the familiar structure of my life disappearing so I am unsure how to be in the space that is left. I can't say that I am welcoming this or inviting it in, but the possibility of doing that intrigues me. I really struggle with the idea that cancer has been sent to me for a reason, as a guide.

That is one of the gifts of poetry, I think, to offer a different way of seeing reality that is not didactic or imposed, but an invitation to see things from a different perspective. And it is so helpful to find words that express some of the half-formed, unspoken thoughts that swirl and gather at a time like this. One of my favourite books is Jeanette Winterson's autobiography *Why be happy when you could be normal?* which is a powerful story of how the discovery of words changed her life. She was adopted as a baby and brought up by a strict, religious mother who was often angry with her. There were only six books in the house where she grew up, one of which was a Bible and two of which were commentaries about the Bible. Her mother was suspicious of what books might contain, but Jeanette found them intriguing and liberating. As a child she read books in secret and gradually worked her way alphabetically through the local public library in Accrington starting with A for Austen.

When she was about to be thrown out of her home at the age of 16 for loving a girl, she found a book of verse by TS Eliot and devoured it, sitting on the steps of the library. Somehow the truth it contained penetrated the hurt and confusion she felt and made things bearable. Poetry helped her make sense of what was happening to her, and helped her navigate her way through it.

I have often been too impatient with poetry to allow it to do its work. In my over-busy life, if I do not 'get' a poem instantly I usually move on to the next thing. But in this newly empty house, there will be more room to linger with words. Perhaps that is part of the new delight.

5

Chemotherapy

June and July

THIS is how I went through treatment for cancer. It is not a prescription or a 'how to' manual. It is not an example to judge, either as one to aspire to or one to criticise; cancer is not a competition. So many factors come into play when you are trying to negotiate a life-changing situation like this, and we all respond in our own unique way. Your way will be different to mine, will be different to hers, will be different to his.

So why share it? Because I felt that being diagnosed with cancer plunged me into a different world where I didn't know the rules or how to find my way around. I wanted to hear from people who had been there before me that it would be okay, that they had navigated this disruption and come out the other side. Like a BBC foreign correspondent, I am reporting back on my experience in that strange land in the hope that it helps other people who have been given the same assignment.

* * * * *

I love runs that take the place of bus or train journeys. I had been working in Westminster for the last three years and had made a practice of running to work once a week. I kept a shower kit in the bottom drawer of my desk and I would take my clothes in the day before so I could run with as little as possible in my backpack. I would set off across Ealing Common at 6.30am and run along the Uxbridge Road into central London, past Middle Eastern shopkeepers setting out displays of fruit and veg, and sleepy commuters standing at bus stops.

After Shepherd's Bush my run converged with the route of the Central Line for a mile or so. I would imagine hot tube carriages stuffed with passengers deep below my feet while I ran through Holland Park and Notting Hill, then I would turn right through the leafy green of Kensington Gardens and Hyde Park. I loved the fact that for two of the last three miles I could run on grass or paths of packed earth, even in the middle of this dense city. Where I could, I would make plans to run to other places, particularly when I was marathon training and needed to fit in high mileage weeks.

A few weeks before my diagnosis I had had a board meeting at Tearfund, a charity I was trustee of. It is based in Teddington, a tedious hour-long bus and train ride away from me. The night before I dropped my clothes off with a friend who works there so she could take them in for me. And then instead of a passive journey on public transport, I ran along the river from Kew, through Richmond to Teddington Lock.

It was a misty morning with the sun just breaking through. There were rowers on the river and herons keeping watch. I shared the path with dog walkers and cyclists, and parents taking children to school. The air was rich with the smell of earth, and I splashed through puddles and squelched through mud. And every moment I felt alive and alert, completely present, aware and slightly in awe of the strength of my body. It enabled me to bring my best self to that meeting.

So, faced with a multitude of hospital appointments over the next few weeks, I had decided to run to those that I could. I had been encouraged when Dr Lewanski had given me the go-ahead to run during chemo, but I didn't know yet how it was going to make me feel, or what impact it would have longer-term on my running. I had been searching online for how other runners had coped with cancer but had found very little information. I wanted to squeeze in as many runs as I could just in case my running was going to be taken away from me.

The day after getting back from Amsterdam, I ran to Charing Cross Hospital for my blood tests and sat outside in the sunshine for a while before going in. It was strange to feel so fit and healthy, having just had such an active weekend, and to know that this building was going to take that away over the next few months. Two days later I did the same again, this time running to my first chemotherapy appointment. I chose to run along the river rather than going the most direct route down the Chiswick High Road; it was longer but more scenic.

From my house, the first couple of miles took me through the peaceful green of Gunnersbury Park and under the M4 to Kew Bridge. I joined the path along the south side of the river, and ran past tennis courts and allotments, alongside rowers and cyclists, under several bridges and beneath canopies of green leaves shimmering in the breeze. Hammersmith Bridge was my cue to cross the river and a couple of hundred metres later I arrived at the hospital. The seven miles was enough time for the anxious tangle of thoughts I had started out with to settle into the simple enjoyment of running and I met Joel outside the hospital with a smile on my face. I got changed in the toilets and we went to find the chemotherapy ward.

But it is a nerve-wracking experience to offer yourself up for treatment that is going to make you unwell in the hope that ultimately it is going to make you better. Doctors have to prepare you for the worst so you hear in great detail all the nastiest side-effects that could be coming your way. We have all heard stories too, whether from friends who have been through it or people in the public eye, about the sickness, fatigue, mental fog, hair loss and so on that usually accompanies chemotherapy. I felt incredibly vulnerable as the nurse, Carly, introduced herself and told us what was about to happen. I was sent for an ECG to check my heart was okay, and Joel and I were shown a DVD about the risk of infection when my blood count would be low after each treatment. Each of these activities prolonged the moment that I was both dreading and desperate for at the same time.

After weeks of talking about chemotherapy, I just wanted to get on with it. Finally, I was shown to a chair in the chemo ward and Joel settled in beside me, a calming presence in such an anxious context. Carly put a drip in the back of my hand and flushed it through with saline solution. My head swam alarmingly and I nearly fainted. How embarrassing; if I couldn't cope with a bit of salt and water, what was going to happen when I was given the strong stuff? Joel fanned my face while I went hot and cold and ten minutes later I was feeling more normal. Anti-sickness medication was next down the line into my bloodstream, followed by three different drugs, one after the other. Carly kept a close eye on me, while Joel gave me a bag of presents from him and Kat. Opening them brought a few minutes' welcome distraction from what was happening. I tried to stay relaxed but it was difficult with the knowledge that I had toxic chemicals entering my body.

Two hours later, I was sent on my way laden down with medication: painkillers, anti-sickness tablets and injections that I would have to give myself in the abdomen over the next week to boost my immune system. We got the tube home and I waited for the drugs to have an effect. That evening and when I woke up in the night I found myself talking to my body as if it were a small child, telling it to be calm, not to feel attacked, to let the drugs do their work, that it will recover, that it will all be okay, that you can do this.

The next morning, I lay in bed and took stock. I had felt a bit nauseous in the night and wired, like I had drunk too much coffee. I went through a mental checklist of different parts of my body to see how they were. I was aware that it would be easy to talk myself into feeling ill because I was waiting for it to happen, and questioning every twinge or bit of tension in my body. But for now I felt okay, so I put on my trainers and went out for a run. I avoided my usual routes, recognising that I didn't need the pressure of comparing this run to my normal pace, and meandered slowly through Ealing's parks and back home.

That afternoon, Jonny drove us down to North Devon, to spend the weekend with our sister-in-law Susie and the rest of his family as part of her 40th birthday celebrations. This weekend away had been in the diary for several months and I didn't want to miss it even though it was so close to my first treatment. Steve, Jonny's brother, and Susie live in Pickwell Manor, a grade II-listed manor house that they share with their friends Tracey and Richard Elliott, and which they also run as a business, renting out the flats on the upper floor as holiday lets and hosting weddings in the ballroom. Steve has an entrepreneurial flair that had enabled him to spot the potential of the manor when they had been in the area on holiday one year. They had worked really hard to make it a success and it was an amazing place to visit when the family all got together.

Susie had organised for everyone to do an assault course at a nearby beach on the Saturday. I had to watch as most of the family struggled into wetsuits and then splashed around on inflatables in the sea. Normally I would have thrown myself into it. Instead I was watching from the sidelines, still waiting for the chemo to take effect, not sure if I could trust how I was feeling or what I could expect of myself at the moment.

Two days later I did start to feel rough, a flu-like, hungover feeling with stomach ache, constipation and nausea. Back home, the next few days sunk into a pattern of feeling restless and uncomfortable, walking slowly to the allotment to pick strawberries or weed half-heartedly, and then coming back home to rest. It was hard to settle in to anything, to concentrate for any length of time.

I invited my mum and Mandy for lunch a week after my first treatment because I knew they wanted to see how I was for myself, but I misjudged how much energy I had and struggled with the simple act of preparing a meal. I was irritable and short-tempered with them, and then felt bad for not being able to cope better. I found myself withdrawing from everyone else, wanting to do this alone, to hibernate away from other people's demands, however well meaning.

I was so grateful for the friends who didn't withdraw from me, who sent cards or messages, welcome communication back from the normal life that I felt was being denied to me. The effect of chemo on my body, mind and soul felt like a prolonged, deep dive under water where the rest of the world was distant, muffled and distorted, and strangely out of reach.

And then, about a week after the treatment, I found myself coming up for air. My stomach settled down, my digestive system was back to normal, my head felt clearer. I went for a run, two slow laps of Ealing Common. It was nothing remarkable. I would normally tag on a lap of the common if I needed to add an extra mile to a longer run rather than it being the main focus. But I was delighted to find that I could still do this, to get back this part of my life that was so important to me, even though it felt different, tentative and hesitant rather than easy and confident.

I was so grateful to be back running that the next day I went along to the Eagles beginners' group, just to run alongside people who were starting out, wanting to offer encouragement on their transition to being a runner, for them to love this as much as I did. With a return to feeling more normal came a profound sense of gratitude. I was grateful for the opportunity to rest, for a workplace that allowed me to take time off, for all the messages of love and support I was getting. And I was acutely aware of how privileged I was in so many ways. Chris was in Gaza that week with some others visiting the Al-Ahli Hospital to find out how Amos Trust could better support them.

Al-Ahli runs a screening programme for breast cancer but many women do not go for screening until it is too late because of the stigma associated with cancer, and resources to treat it are limited. Their survival rate is 40 per cent ten years on whereas in the UK it is nearly 80 per cent. I was getting excellent medical care for free, could indulge myself with a healthy diet, was enveloped by love from my family and friends, and so in the middle of it all I could honestly say that I was blessed.

In the third week, I was back at work. It was strange to plunge back into a set of concerns and priorities that had carried on without me, while I had been in such a different space. I felt very strongly that work was not a place to be vulnerable. If I was going to turn up there, I needed to be a competent version of myself rather than expecting people to cover for me more than they were already. If I felt wobbly, I decided that I would talk to Jonny rather than confide in my colleagues. But there was also something reassuring about having this part of my life back too. Work generated things that needed to be done, and so I got on with them, caught up again in the normality of it all, grateful to have something to concentrate on that didn't involve hospitals or medicine or treatment plans.

But I was aware that the next chemotherapy was looming, that this respite was only temporary. I wanted to be able to run to hospital again so I ran five miles during the week, and joined my running club at a 10k Summer League race in Harrow that weekend. The Summer League is a series of five or six races hosted by different London running clubs, either five miles or 10k, as well as races for children and relays for the adults. The first time the Eagles had joined in a few years before, there had been around ten of us; now we usually got a huge turnout and it was always a really enjoyable day out in good company.

It was harder than I expected, however, to be content with just running the distance. I watched the people I used to compete with get PBs while I trogged round not racing at all. I knew it was ridiculous to expect my body to perform as normal when it was coping with so much but I couldn't help feeling disappointed with my time of 55:36 – a minute a mile slower than my best. I was re-reading Mark Rowlands's book *Running with the Pack,* philosophical observations on running and life that resonated deeply with me. He talks about discovering the intrinsic value of running, not to race or achieve or compete. You don't need reasons to run when you are a kid or a dog, he reminds us. In the past, I had run to expand my horizons, to discover what I was capable of, to give myself headspace, to be my best self.

Perhaps now my running needed to shift to running for the simple joy of it, to feel alive, to stay connected to who I have been, to find a new normal, to celebrate this imperfect body that was coping with so much.

Monday was my last day at work in that first cycle of treatment and I met up with a friend for a meal in the evening, wanting to squeeze every last moment of normality out of the day. On Tuesday I went back to Charing Cross Hospital for blood tests in the morning, and spent the remainder of the day restless and out of sorts. Having been through my first chemo treatment, I think I expected the second one to be a breeze but as it approached I found myself getting more and more apprehensive about entering 'cancer world' again. I slept really badly that night, getting up in the small hours to drink tea in the kitchen rather than lying sleepless in bed. On Wednesday morning, I paced around the house waiting for my appointment, weighed down with sadness and a deep sense of grief. I found it impossible to shake off these dark feelings. It felt as though they were physically present, silent beings lingering just outside my line of vision.

Perhaps inspired by the poem Grace had given me for my birthday, I found myself naming them as sorrow, loss, loneliness and helplessness, and then welcoming them into the room, inviting them to sit with me for a while, asking them what I needed to learn from them; what did they have to teach me? Tears flowed as the feelings overwhelmed me but it felt important to let them, not to pretend that I was okay, but to acknowledge every way in which this cancer experience was affecting me.

And then it was time to set off for hospital. I had arranged to run there with Lucy Rigg. She was a teacher who worked four days a week, and whose free day was Wednesday, very conveniently the same day as my treatments. I had first got to know her a couple of years before when she had joined the beginners' group that Mark and I were leading. She had quickly progressed from a 5k to 10k, and on to the Ealing Half-Marathon six months later, and the previous year I had written her a training plan for the London Marathon, where she had easily finished in under four hours.

Lucy has a slight Glaswegian twang from her childhood growing up in Scotland, and is a wonderfully easy person to be with. A run with her always involves an interesting conversation at the same time, and I knew that she would be good company on this particular journey. I left my house to meet her on the way, still weighed down with sadness. I muttered as I ran, 'Okay sorrow, you can come with me but you're going to have to keep up.' Lucy was waiting for me in the park and we set off towards Kew Bridge.

And that run was just what I needed. As we ran along the river, I felt the weight of sadness lift off my shoulders, almost like a physical release. The familiar rhythm of my feet on the path soothed me, and Lucy's company lifted my spirits. I ran more slowly than the previous time, but the fact that I was repeating the same route held the promise that I would bounce back from this season, that cancer would not have the last word.

I drank in the beauty of the trees along the route, the calm of the river, the smell of the earth we were running on, packed hard by so many people making this same journey. Once again, I experienced the untangling effect of running, of it drawing my thoughts away from the fear and anxiety about what lay ahead into the intensity of the present moment. All that was needed was being here, the synchronisation of breath, arms and feet carrying us along. I wanted to run on and on but all too soon, Hammersmith Bridge came into view. We crossed the river and arrived at the hospital a few minutes later, to meet Jonny who had fresh clothes for me in a bag. I hugged Lucy goodbye, and walked into the building feeling so much lighter than when I had set out.

Cancer laughs in the face of any plans you try to make, but that run made me even more determined to run to all my chemotherapy appointments. If the river route proved to be too long, I would take a different way. Even if I had to get the tube part of the way and only jog the final few yards to the hospital, I wanted to arrive in my trainers and on my terms.

I got changed and we went to wait for a free chair in the chemo ward. And then after the high of my run, the cancer rollercoaster took a downward plunge. My doctor had not signed off on my treatment after my blood tests the day prior, an essential step before the chemo nurse could access the drugs I would need. It took them over an hour to get her approval, and then when I did get settled in a chair, bracing myself for the drip to be inserted in my hand, I was told that I would only be getting one of the drugs that day instead of all three.

The blood tests showed that my liver and kidneys were not functioning very well; the level of one particular enzyme was three times as high as normal and they were concerned that my body just wasn't coping with the chemotherapy. It was all very confusing. The nurses on the ward couldn't give me any information about what it would mean, because they were just carrying out the registrar's instructions.

Rather than feeling relief that I was getting a lighter dose of chemo, I was deeply disappointed. I didn't know if this meant that I would have to have an extra treatment later on, prolonging the chemo and delaying surgery. Or whether this meant the cancer was less treatable and therefore more serious. Ridiculous as this may sound, I felt as though I was failing somehow and I wondered if I had done something wrong. Tears rolled down my face as the drug dripped into my veins and I returned home weighed down and anxious.

My mum arrived that afternoon and stayed for a couple of days. She and my dad, Ian, had been childhood sweethearts who had been married for over 50 years, and they had done everything together, my dad leading the way and my mum happily following him. Towards the end of my dad's life, he had got steadily more frail and my mum's world had got smaller as she devoted herself to looking after him. For the last two years of his life he was confined to bed and her world became their house and garden, with occasional trips to the shops. At the time, it seemed to me that what was happening to him was the mirror image of the start in life that he and my mum had given to me.

There is something very mysterious about a newborn baby, so much of her character and personality are yet to be discovered. As you nurture your child there is an unfolding and a revealing of who they are; you watch in delight as they become themselves, as they explore the world, as they need you less, as they grow away. The future is heavy with potential and possibilities; everything is ahead and there is so much to look forward to. On my dad's journey to death there was a drawing in, a needing more, a silencing of a once-strong voice, a diluting of a dominant personality. There was sadness at what was being lost and a deep gratitude for all that had been. In those last few months of his life, everything was behind us.

Without knowing it at the time, I had had my best conversations with him. I had survived our worst misunderstanding. We had shared our deepest belly laughs. I had had my last hug. My dad believed in a life after this one, but even so we were heading back into mystery and unknowing, into a place beyond language.

Much as I loved my dad, my prayer for him was for a good end to his life that would not be prolonged. I found the liminal space of his frailty and his neediness too uncomfortable and I wanted it to be over. I watched my mum with awe. She had bound her life to his for over 50 years. She had the tenacity and tenderness to walk this final stage with him with dignity and respect, and always with love. I hoped that if the same thing was required of me one day that I would offer it with the same willingness and grace.

My sisters and I did what we could in that season to help from a distance and each of us took on different roles. My youngest sister Susie provided most of the practical and emotional support that mum needed because she lived in the same town and called in to see them most days. I became the one who sorted things out, who got a blue disabled badge for their car, who arranged for a stairlift to be installed in their house. After my dad died, I kept trying to fix things, wanting to help my mum make the most of this next stage of her life. I encouraged her to get her fitness back by going for regular walks, and took her a passport application form to fill in.

My dad had done National Service in Cyprus and Egypt when he was younger and that seemed to have put him off travelling abroad; almost all of our holidays had been in caravan sites in

England or Wales and my mum had never left the country. Once she had her passport, Mandy and I took her to Germany for the weekend to visit Harry on his year abroad in Hanover. Now, having her to stay when I was ill, our relationship shifted again. I couldn't fix anything about what was happening to me, and nor could she. She was just there for me, happy to do mundane things like washing up and watching TV, simply wanting to play a part in what I was going through, and it was very comforting to have her with me.

I e-mailed my breast cancer nurse, Nikki, my point of contact with my medical team, to find out more about the implications of missing some of the chemotherapy drugs and she promised to investigate for me. Having done the dive into a chemo haze once, I knew what to expect and for the next couple of days I enjoyed spending time with my mum, walking to the shops to buy fruit and veg, and pottering around the allotment picking strawberries and raspberries. The weekend brought the same slide into feeling ill as before, a heavy woolliness descending on my body and my mind, slowing me down and distracting my thoughts.

I felt spaced out and fuzzy-headed. I got fixated on my digestive system, trying to gauge how much lactulose to take to stop myself getting too constipated, trying to find healthy things to eat when I had little appetite so that I didn't lose too much weight. My feelings seemed to be under the same heavy cloud; it was difficult to feel enthusiastic about anything, or to feel much at all really.

Once again I hid myself away from other people, lacking the energy to arrange anything and not knowing how to be myself with others while I felt like this. I went out for a walk each day to get out of the house. I felt like I had turned into an 80-year-old version of myself, staying close to home, the highlight of my day being an amble to the shops before coming back to watch *Pointless* on TV. Nikki got back in touch but didn't have much information; her advice was to wait until I saw the registrar when I had my next set of blood tests before my third chemo treatment. I would just have to be patient.

Then on the Monday, five days after my second treatment, the fog began to lift. Having just one drug was obviously a lot easier for my body to deal with. So I went for a run, my instinctive response to feeling more normal. I did a simple two laps of Ealing Common again, but it was so good to be out and active. I felt like all my senses were heightened after those few days of feeling muffled and deadened. There was heavy traffic on the North Circular which cuts across the common but even here I ran on a trail, through long, wet grass, breathing in the cool smell of damp earth after the overnight rain. It was a slow, tentative run but in my head I was saying to myself, 'Look, I'm running!' and it did my soul good.

Back at home I was still buzzing as I had a shower and ate breakfast. I have always been a better evangelist for running than I ever was for Jesus. I wanted to say to everyone I met: go running while you can (or if running is not your thing, then swim, cycle, walk, box). Get your heart pumping and your lungs working. Use your body, push yourself beyond your limits, feel the sweet ache of muscles that have worked hard and are letting you know about it. Get off the treadmill and out of the gym. Run in the rain, in the shade, in the sun. Run through parks, along canals, beside roads, on trails. Run for your life, and your life will thank you for it.

Now I felt more myself, I rang the hospital and spoke to my registrar about my liver. She was reassuring but could not say for definite what it would mean in terms of treatment. They would monitor how my body was responding and adjust things accordingly. It did not necessarily mean that I would have to have an extra chemotherapy session. The fact that the chemo had hit my body so hard meant that it was hitting the cancer hard too, and if I couldn't cope with the drugs they would do the surgery earlier. It made me realise how much I like a plan, to know what was going to happen when, and I found it really unsettling to have things change around me.

Once again I tried to stay with what I knew, to be in the moment, rather than letting the anxiety about what might be ahead take over. I made the most of the chemo fog receding and met up with friends for coffee or lunch; just doing one thing each day made me feel more normal.

My sense of identity was being seriously challenged by having cancer. Throughout my life I had experienced moments of self-doubt and a sometimes crippling lack of confidence, but generally, having reached 50, I felt competent at work, I enjoyed a sense of achievement in my running and I felt at home in my community of friends. Now all of that seemed to be shifting. Work felt far less significant because I was not there very much at the moment. I wasn't sure what my body was capable of any more, whether I should be resting more or whether it was okay to try and run as much as possible, whether a run would be energising or add to my fatigue.

My relationships felt in flux too; some people I had expected to support me were keeping their distance, while other people that I hardly knew had drawn close and been wonderfully caring. That sense of movement all around me wasn't necessarily a negative thing, but it did make me feel vulnerable and insecure which I found unsettling. I was not sure how to respond. I didn't want to let the vulnerability and weakness dominate so that I wore them as a badge and ended up feeling incompetent and unable, but neither did I want to toughen up and try to carry on as before which felt as though I would be missing an invitation to grow through this whole experience.

I wanted to find a third way, to acknowledge the frailty I felt but not let it define me, to draw on a deeper sense of self and to stay connected to all that I had been up to this point so that I could be my true self in this difficult time. Frailty and vulnerability are not the same as learned helplessness and passivity. I realised that I could be weak and vulnerable and still have agency. I could choose how I responded.

And sometimes my response was to get angry. On Friday, ten days after my second chemo, I woke up in a bad mood. I was so tired of being careful to avoid infections, of taking things easy in case I wore myself out, of looking strange because I was bald, of not being able to make plans, of being passive and having things done to me. I put on my trainers and went out for a run. Instead of the slow amble round the parks that I had been doing, I headed down to the river to get in a few more miles. Instead of being tentative I picked up the pace. The mantra in my head as I ran was, 'Fuck off cancer. Fuck off self-pity.' My feet pounded the pavement and I arrived home out of breath but more at peace. It was a cathartic and energising run – just what I needed.

That weekend I went to lectures for the MSc I was doing in voluntary sector management at Cass Business School. I was studying alongside my work and I was in the second year with just two modules to go. Technically, I could have asked for a year off because I had a serious illness and then returned to finish it in 2016, but with relatively little left to do I wanted to continue if I could. I had really enjoyed the study the year before and had made a good group of friends from the Action Learning Set I had been put in.

There had been a weekend of the course six weeks previously, just after I had got my diagnosis. I hadn't told people about the cancer then, partly because it was so new and I was just coming to terms with it and partly because it was hard to know how to drop it into the conversation. I didn't want to talk about it when I first met people because I didn't want to dominate things, but by the end of the day it got harder to bring it up because I hadn't mentioned it before. Instead I had e-mailed my closest friends on the course afterwards and they were all incredibly supportive. The last two modules were on grant making and philanthropy and over the next few weeks I would need to do an essay and an exam. Claire Angus, a super-efficient, down-to-earth Canadian accountant, arranged some Skype revision sessions with a small group of us, so that they could share with me what they were researching. I was very touched.

And then the next week I was back to work again. I felt stronger than I had done at the same point in the previous cycle and I had run over 20 miles in the last week, which showed how much easier it had been for my body to cope with just one drug. I went up to Liverpool for a couple of days to host a gathering of the network of organisations that I manage. People were pleased to see me, and very kind. It was a gorgeously hot week in June and I was quite glad the hotel we were in had the air-conditioning turned up which meant I needed to keep my beanie hat on otherwise I was too cold; I was too self-conscious to be bald in front of my wider network of colleagues, some of whom I didn't know very well and all of whom I needed to work professionally with.

Secretly, I was starting to think about the running I wanted to do in the months to come. I knew by now that making firm plans would be difficult until my treatment was over, so instead I tried to create possibilities, a small but subtle distinction that helped me hold these ideas more lightly and cope better if and when I had to let go of them. On the Friday, I ran nearly ten miles before work. Looking ahead, my last chemo treatment was due three weeks before the Ealing Half-Marathon. I had been a pacer for the first two years of the race and had had to miss it the previous year because of a twisted ankle. I wondered if I might be able to do it this year.

I didn't know what state I would be in at the end of chemotherapy, but I decided that if I could run ten miles in between each cycle, then I could make it round the 13.1 miles of the course even if I did it very slowly. I also signed up for the 2016 London Marathon using my good-for-age time from the Chester Marathon the previous October. I thought it would be a great way to celebrate the end of my treatment for cancer if I was up to it by then, and I needed to enter the race now if I was to have any chance of doing it.

It was time for treatment number three. On Monday I had blood taken, and then went to see Dr Lewanski the next day to find out what my liver was doing. The enzyme levels were still a lot higher than normal, but not as dramatically as the previous time, and I could have all three drugs again in this cycle of treatment. The single drug had not really reduced the size of the tumour so there was no point just having one. They would keep monitoring me carefully and if my liver function got worse again, they would perform the surgery earlier.

We talked about my alcohol consumption and he told me that the half a bottle of wine I often enjoyed three or four times a week put me in the binge-drinking category which was literally rather sobering. I love wine and I find it really hard to just have one glass. Seasons of training for marathons had been a helpful way for me to cut down on my alcohol intake over the last few years. I would choose not to drink alcohol if I was going to be running the next day which meant I only had wine once or twice a week but I wasn't always that disciplined. I decided not to drink for the rest of my chemotherapy but knew I also needed to cut down permanently.

That evening I felt vulnerable and sad again, but not as low as the previous time. I tried to acknowledge the sadness without indulging in self-pity. And I had arranged my run to hospital ahead of time. Lucy was coming with me again, and Christine Elliott was going to join us.

Chris is a journalist at BBC News Online and an Eagle who got similar times in races to me, usually a bit faster. She had finished her first marathon in Manchester in under four hours in 2012 which had given me hope at the time that I would one day do the same thing. Harry was running with us too, and was going to sit with me through the chemo treatment. He hadn't done much running since the London Marathon a few months before, and he was going to be weighed down by my bag of clothes to change into but that didn't seem to bother him.

My sister Liz had texted me the night before, to ask what time we were going to be running. She was planning to go and run beside her local river at the same time, so she would be with us in spirit. Liz is only 16 months older than me. My mum dressed us identically when we were little, in clothes that she made for us herself, and as I was big for my age and Liz was small for hers, people had often thought we were twins. We had shared a bedroom for most of our childhood and teenage years, and had paired up as the 'big ones' in contrast to my two younger sisters. At secondary school we had often been mistaken for each other, and I remember getting intensely annoyed when my English teacher wrote 'well done Liz' in my exercise book.

We had been very close when we were growing up but had seen less of each other as adults for the simple reason that we were all busy with our own lives and children. I was really touched that she wanted to be part of my chemo run, that she was stepping into this space with me.

At the time, the act of running to hospital completely reframed what was going on. Instead of dreading the treatment, I looked forward to the run. Having people to run with meant I felt safe; if it had proved too much for me they would have made sure I was all right. I would never have run there alone, and I don't know if they realised at the time what a gift they were giving me by enabling me to run. Getting to the hospital on my own feet gave me a feeling of agency and almost a sense of power, to be doing something on my terms that was completely disconnected to the world of ill health that I was reluctantly inhabiting. Cancer had taken so many things from me; it was not having this.

Looking back, memories of that run are of sunshine and conversation, light-heartedness and companionship. I smile when I think of us running along that river path even though I know what came next. At the hospital, we waved Lucy and Chris goodbye. Harry came with me to the chemo ward where he was a comforting presence as I offered my arm for the infusion of chemicals.

The next few days followed a by now familiar pattern. My mum came to stay for a while again just to be with me and then I dipped into the twilight world as the drugs took effect. I seemed to feel the most unsettled and apprehensive as I was having the chemo, even though it did not have an immediate impact. That lessened over the next couple of days as there was a surrender to the inevitability of what was to come, a descent into a place of dis-ease and discomfort, of a veil being drawn between my reality and that of everyone else. This time felt harder and it made me realise again how much easier it had been to just have one drug.

Over the next few days my bowels seemed to dominate everything else. I oscillated between constipation and diarrhoea, between taking lactulose and imodium, and never quite getting it right. The journal where I wrote my deepest thoughts descended into a poo diary for a while as I kept track of what my insides were doing. I was restless and bad-tempered. I felt bleurgh; I felt nothingy; I felt weak and ill.

This time there was no joyful two laps of the common a few days after treatment; I had to do the exam for my course ten days later. I was very grateful for the revision session that Claire had organised and I felt like I leant very heavily on my friends without being able to offer anything in return. I tried to read the papers other people had found and was grateful that I could take in a page of notes which meant I didn't need to try and remember anything. It is surprising how many words you can get on one sheet of A4 if you use three columns, tiny margins and a very small font.

I had told the university that I would be in the middle of cancer treatment, and they made welcome concessions. I was able to use a computer instead of writing, and I was allowed rest breaks. The exam was something to endure rather than try to excel at, and I was glad when it was over.

The next day I did a slow jog round the parks and started to feel more normal. A friend, Azariah France-Williams, messaged me to see if I wanted to go and do Wormwood Scrubs parkrun with him on Saturday. Azariah and I had crossed paths many years before when we both worked for the same youth work organisation and I had met him again quite recently through my current job. He was a priest at a church on a housing estate in North Kensington and highly creative, and he and his wife, Anna, had a joyful determination to live life well. We had invited them round for a meal back in May, which turned out to be shortly after my diagnosis. We talked about cancer and death that night, as well as a host of other more normal things, and that seemed to have fast-forwarded our friendship.

I had always been primarily a lone runner. When I started running that was because I didn't know anyone else who ran, but even though I had been in the Eagles for several years, I still did most of my running on my own. That was partly because I like to run first thing in the morning and it is hard to find people who want to set off at 6.30am; partly because running was my headspace and I really enjoyed the solitude and opportunity to just be, to experience what Mark Rowlands calls the 'freedom of spending time with the mind'; and partly because in a marathon you need to draw on your own resources to keep going, and so it made sense to me to get used to that in preparation. I always really appreciated the running I did with other people, especially long runs leading up to marathons, but my default type of running was solitary.

So in this enforced season of running differently, it was good to rediscover the joy of running with other people. A few weeks before, I did Gunnersbury parkrun with Tracey Melville, a friend who had had treatment for cancer the year before and who was a wonderful, hopeful embodiment of the life that will return. Tracey had joined the first beginners' group that Mark and I had run a few years before, and I had loved watching her conquer different distances as her confidence in her running grew. Soon after my diagnosis she invited me round for coffee and had patiently listened to my fears and apprehension, offering the wisdom she had gained from her experience.

At parkrun we jogged slowly round Gunnersbury Park, talking and laughing, oblivious to how fast we were going, just enjoying each other's company. The Saturday after Azariah's text message, I cycled slowly over to Wormwood Scrubs to join him. As we ran, we talked about anything and everything, catching up with each other as we tagged along at the end of the pack of runners. Azariah quoted the African saying, 'If you want to go fast, go alone. If you want to go far, go together.' It seemed a good fit for the season I was in.

It made me realise that I could be quite a solitary person a lot of the time, someone who is self-sufficient, who sorts things out for herself and tends not to ask for help. I had made a conscious decision at the start of all this to accept every comment, message or offer in the spirit in which it was intended and to welcome people into this strange space with me, rather than attempting to do it alone.

Presence is a very powerful thing, to be with someone without needing to fix them or change things, to help them explore their reality without telling them what to do or how to do it, to go at their pace, not yours. Presence does not even have to be physical; there were people who I knew were with me even though I hadn't seen them since this began. Running with Azariah round Wormwood Scrubs was an embodiment of all the different ways people were with me.

And he always asks me good questions. When he and Anna came round for a meal, he had asked me if I had a metaphor for the way I thought about cancer. Was it an adversary that I was battling against, or a companion that I would journey with for a while? It is a good question and one that I had thought about a lot since. When you are facing something unknown, a metaphor can help you get your head round what is happening and provide a way in to thinking about it. A metaphor is never perfect, but it can set your thoughts in the right direction and bring the unknown into reach.

There is divided opinion about using the metaphor of fighting or battling with cancer. It seems to me that it is most often used by people who are looking on, to describe what they see their friends and family going through and used far less by people who have cancer themselves. As I have said, I found it hard to get my head around the fact that this cancer was not something alien that had invaded my body, it was my own cells that had gone haywire, that were out of control. This tumour was a part of me, and while I hadn't got to the point of welcoming it and I was keen to get rid of it, I didn't want to plunge myself into civil war where I was raging against my own body.

I had battled enough against a fierce inner critic for many years who had tried to wear me down with an internal monologue of all the ways in which I was deficient; this was a season for being kind to myself. And I didn't feel like I was fighting for my life. This cancer was treatable, and although it felt more serious now that I knew my liver was suffering, and I knew there was always a possibility that I will look back on these words with regret, my attitude was that I had some unpleasant months to go through and then it would be over.

In many ways it seemed to me that this cancer was more like a hostile lodger that you rented your spare room to, and you are now locked into a contract that you can't end early. She arrived with good references and seemed nice when you first met her, but after a few pleasant months when you hardly noticed she was there, she has turned into the lodger from hell, disrupting your sleep with late night noise, being rude when friends come round, leaving washing-up to fester in the kitchen and filling your home with tension and dread. Even when you don't see much of her, her malevolent presence cannot be ignored and the process of getting rid of her just makes everything worse.

How did you let someone so nasty into your home which should be a sanctuary and a place of safety? But although she may leave you without paying her rent, with a room that needs completely redecorating, and with a less naïve approach to sharing your space, she will be gone in the near future, and your home will be your own once more.

But perhaps unsurprisingly the metaphor that most resonated was still that of training for an endurance event. I was nearly halfway through my 18-week plan, and my surgery was booked for October with a period of recovery afterwards. My badly functioning liver was like a sprained ankle that was slowing my progress but didn't mean I was out of the race yet. I was ticking off the weeks one by one, enjoying some and enduring others. It was a slow slog that I was finding hard, but one that was falling into a recognisable pattern, and there was an end in sight.

Sadly, I was about to discover that there was still a lot to get through before the end. The next day I noticed that my left arm, where I had had my last chemo infusion, was badly swollen, and it had a hard lump on the inside just above my elbow. My left hand was noticeably fatter than my right. I didn't know if it was anything to worry about; perhaps I had been bitten by something?

I rang the out-of-hours number for the chemo ward but wasn't able to get through. We were going over to Joel and Kat's for lunch and I was desperate for some fun and normality so I put it out of my mind and just enjoyed the day.

On Monday we drove to Bristol for Harry's graduation. Joel had got a degree in graphic design and communication three years before from Chelsea Art College, but hadn't wanted to go to his graduation and so we missed it too. I was very keen to be there for Harry's, my one chance to be a proud parent at a graduation ceremony.

I was worried about the state of my arm, however; it had got worse overnight instead of better and was now red and even more swollen. While we were waiting to go into the graduation hall I rang the chemo ward again and got through this time. I spoke to Rosie, the nurse who had done my last two treatments, and she told me to go straight to A&E for an ultrasound. Bristol Royal Infirmary was just down the road so while Jonny watched Harry graduating, I sat in a joyless waiting room with a too-loud TV blaring out frantic dance music. They did blood tests and ended up giving me antibiotics several hours later, saying that it was probably cellulitis from an insect bite.

Harry had found a vegan restaurant where we could have a celebratory lunch, but there was no time to get there and instead we had pizza in a microbrewery across the road from where he graduated. It was fine but not the way I would have chosen to mark his graduation and I felt that the attention had been on me rather than on Harry who deserved to be in the limelight.

The following day I was back at work again. It was a tough week. I was feeling sorry for myself because of my arm, and it was hard to address things properly in just a few days. Some members of my team were overloaded because they were picking up my work as well as their own and they were feeling the strain. All I could do was listen as they offloaded and try to suggest ways to deal with it. They were not blaming me, and it was my job to support them but it was hard not to feel guilty at what I was putting them through.

Bethany, one of my colleagues, gave me a hug as I was leaving one day and I cried all the way home; that small act of compassion unlocked how I was really feeling. By Friday my arm still wasn't any better, so I rang the hospital again and spent the day at Charing Cross Hospital. They were concerned that the swelling might be caused by blood clots so I had to wait several hours for an ultrasound. Fortunately that was all clear and they agreed that the antibiotics I had been given at BRI were what I needed. Eventually they let me out in time to meet my family and go to the theatre, a long-planned treat to celebrate Harry's graduation. It had been a frustrating few days; lots of activity and lots of waiting around but nothing to show for any of it.

That weekend I ran ten miles, in spite of my swollen arm, still holding on to the dream of doing Ealing Half, still determined to stay on my feet and not descend into despair. I was weak and weary but I was nearly halfway through and I was not going to be beaten.

Rediscovering Writing

There are some stories about cancer that are utterly tragic and justify the fear and dread that swirl around the word. I think Kate Gross's story is one of those. She was a high-flyer who worked for two prime ministers in her 20s. Aged 30, she was CEO of the African Governance Initiative, working with fragile democracies across the continent. She was married with twin boys. Then when she was 34, she was diagnosed with bowel cancer after it had spread to her liver. She died two years later on Christmas Eve, just before her boys came down to open their stockings.

Kate wrote a blog while she had cancer, and then wrote a book, *Late Fragments*, for The Knights, as she called her boys, so that they would understand more about who she was when they grew up. It is a beautifully written book about life and how to live it well. She finds a sense of clarity and wholeness among the pain and loss in the months leading up to her death. And one of the things that contributes to that is rediscovering the joy of writing, something she had loved as a child, but that had got squeezed out in the busyness of her life. She writes:

'I wonder whether this unexpected sense of completeness stems from something else, something which applies as much to you lucky sods who have decades ahead of you. I'm not doing what I was before, but I am not doing nothing. I am writing. The clickety-clack of my fingers on the keyboard is like the sound of rain on parched fields. Why did I ever stop doing this? If words are who I am, how did I let this become such a marginal part of my life?

'You know the answer because I have described my neglected hinterland. It happens: work is, for most of us, what we do with our outer selves, the grown-up tip of the iceberg that we show the world, which takes up our time and energy. But in all that aching and striving and achieving it is so easy to lose sight of the things which truly define us. These things try to break through, insistently, because they matter.'

I can so identify with her words. I earned my living from writing for 12 years, wrote an award-winning charity blog for five years, have written lots of youth work resources and one proper book, and yet you can see from this blog how intermittent that writing had become. I had little to write about and no time to write it. Cancer has given me back that desire to write to try and make sense of what is happening to me.

I write in my previously neglected journal every day, sometimes two or three times, and you get the edited highlights here. I write in my journal the things that I can't even say to anyone else, the darkest thoughts, and then I look back the next day and realise that I have moved on, that things are not that bad, but that somehow putting them into words and writing them down released their power over me.

And writing here has stripped away the sense of isolation that I felt when I first heard my diagnosis. Early on I wrote in my journal, 'Cancer turns you into an exhibit. You slip into a parallel world where things are not what they were and people observe you with pity to see how you are coping.'

I still feel sometimes like I am in a completely different space, but I know that so many people have entered that space with me rather than watching from a distance. We all struggle with what to say when people we love face something like this and I am so grateful for every comment here and on social media in response to what I write, and all the e-mails, texts and phone calls. Everyone has to deal with cancer in the way that suits them and not everyone chooses to do it in public. But this suits me and has led to the most amazing conversations and connections with people.

Cancer has disrupted my plans, my sense of identity, my knowledge of what I am physically capable of, and my place in the world but it has also given me back the desire and the time to write and for that I am hugely grateful. It has shown me that people love me more than I ever knew. I have found going back into the second round of treatment really hard, but I know I am not alone and that means the world to me.

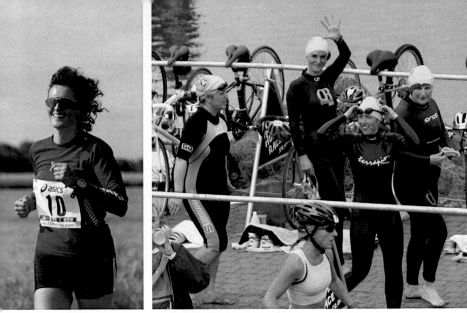

Run section of an Olympic distance triathlon at Dorney Lake, September 2007. **Photo: Jonny Baker**

Waving just before the swim in a sprint distance triathlon at Dorney Lake, June 2007.
Photo: Jonny Baker

My mum and my sisters: Liz Low, Mary Slark, Susie Stanforth, Mandy Keasley and me. **Photo: Jonny Baker**

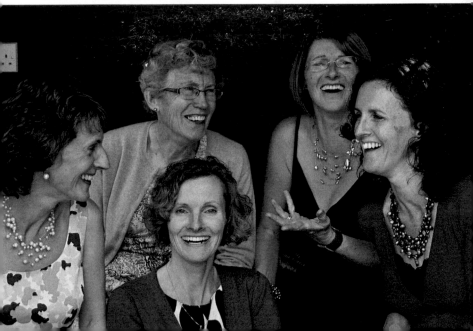

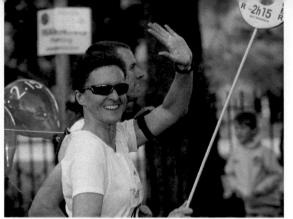

Pacing 2 hours 15 at the first Ealing Half-Marathon with Flatfoot Dave. **Photo: Jonny Baker**

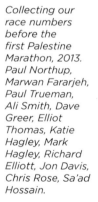

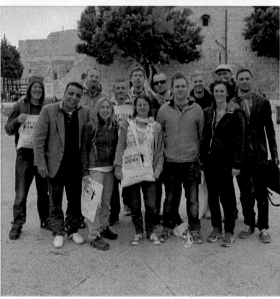

Collecting our race numbers before the first Palestine Marathon, 2013. Paul Northup, Marwan Fararjeh, Paul Trueman, Ali Smith, Dave Greer, Elliot Thomas, Katie Hagley, Mark Hagley, Richard Elliott, Jon Davis, Chris Rose, Sa'ad Hossain.

Paul Trueman, Sa'ad Hossain, Jon David, Jenny Baker, Elliot Thomas, Bob Mayo, Paul Northup, Mark Hagley, Katie Hagley, Dave Greer, Richard Elliott, Ali Smith. **Photo: Chris Rose**

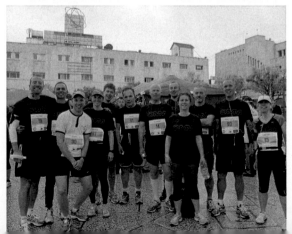

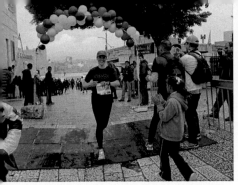

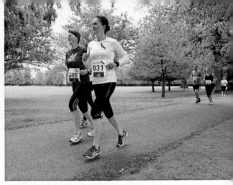

Crossing the finish line at the first Palestine Marathon.

Pacing my sister Mandy to a PB, Ealing Eagles 10k, 2013. **Photo: Kieren Geaney**

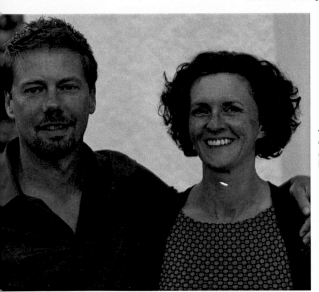

Jonny and Jenny Baker, on holiday in Pembrokeshire, 2014. **Photo: Harry Baker**

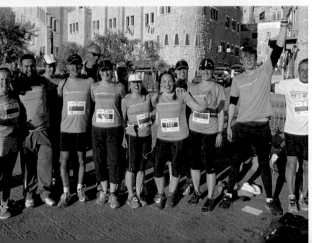

At the second Palestine Marathon, ready to run. Philippa Stroud, Asad Kayani, Jack Rose, Matt Crisp, Chris Rose, Susie Baker, Toria Moore, Ali Smith, Jaqs Waggett, Tracey Elliott, Jenny Baker, David Smith, Paul Sanderson.

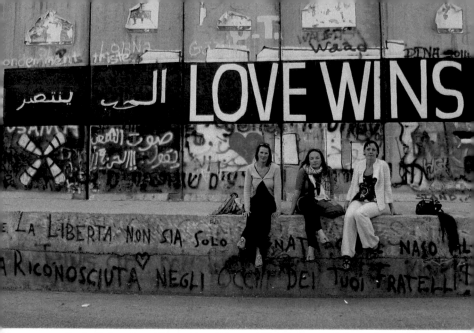

Susie Baker, Jaqs Waggett and Tracey Elliott in front of the wall, Bethlehem, 2014. **Photo: Jenny Baker**

With the remains of my black eye in Manger Square, and Mandy Keasley, 2015. **Photo: Grace Wroe**

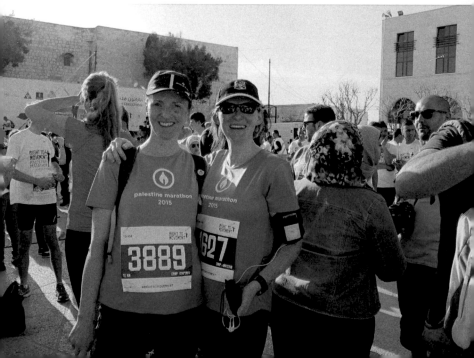

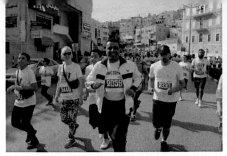

Marwan Fararjeh running the 10k, 2015.
Photo: Jenny Baker

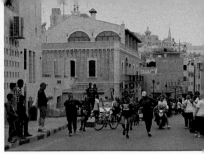

Nader al-Masri about to win the 2015 Palestine Marathon.
Photo: Jenny Baker

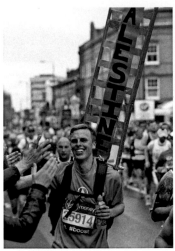

Harry Baker running the London Marathon, 2015. **Photo: Jonny Baker**

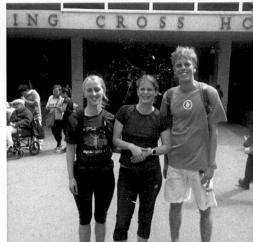

Christine Elliott, Lucy Rigg, Harry Baker, Charing Cross Hospital. Round three of chemo, July 2015. **Photo: Jenny Baker**

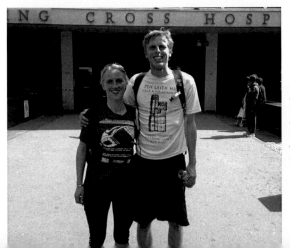

Christine Elliott, Harry Baker, Charing Cross Hospital. Round four of chemo, July 2015. **Photo: Jenny Baker**

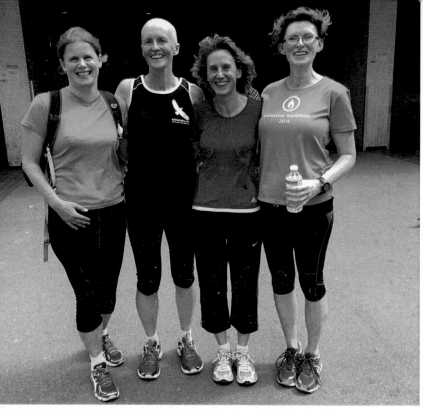

Lucy Rigg, Jenny Baker, Liz Low, Mandy Keasley, Charing Cross Hospital. Run to port fitting, August 2015.

Lucy Rigg, Mandy Keasley, Joel Baker, Harry Baker, me, Neil Enskat, Charing Cross Hospital, September 2015. Final round of chemo.

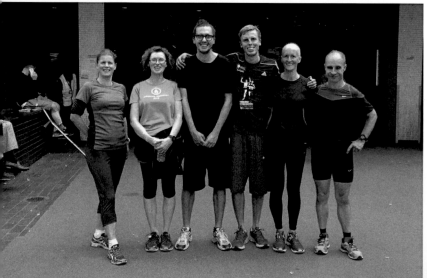

Me and Jon Birch, Bath,
August 2015.
Photo: Jonny Baker

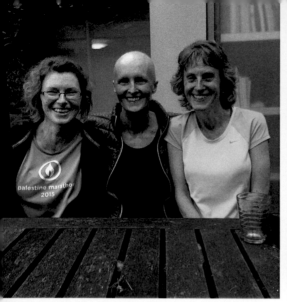

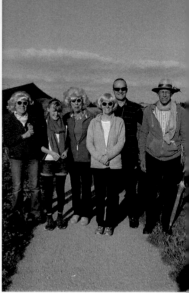

Mandy Keasley, me and Liz Low, having lunch in the Maggie's Centre, Charing Cross, just before final chemo, September 2015. **Photo: Joel Baker**

Mary Slark, Carrie Stanforth, Meg Payne, Susie Stanforth, Dave Stanforth and John Payne, walking along the river in Ely in solidarity with my final chemo run, September 2015. **Photo: Jacob Stanforth**

Me and Florence, Greenwich, October 2015. **Photo: Jonny Baker**

My hair growing back, Pickwell, November 2015. **Photo: Jonny Baker**

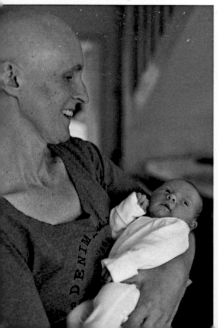

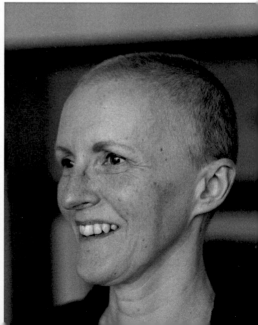

6

Losing My Hair

June to November

MANY women can tell you stories about their hair – about the disastrous haircut or the misjudged perm; about the joy of finding a hairdresser who cuts it just right and the lengths we will go to stick with her; about the thin line between loving how you look and another bad hair day; about how a bit of rain can turn your sleek curls into unmanageable frizz. I have all those stories and more.

However much we might want to be free from the pressure of always looking presentable, what we look like does matter and hair is a huge factor in looking good.

It might sound bizarre but it took me ages to appreciate that I had curly hair. As a child I had it cut in a pageboy and my mum would blow it dry and curl the ends under. In my teens I hated my hair and spent hours trying to control it. It was the 1980s and I could have had the trendy 'shaggy perm' style without the bother of perming it, but I spent an inordinate amount of time trying to get my hair to 'flick' at the sides instead.

This was in the days before hair straighteners and I used clips to try and keep it in place. I would position my hair very carefully when I put my head on my pillow at night, and I even went through a phase of wearing a bobble hat as it dried in a vain attempt to achieve the smooth and silky look I craved.

A new hairdresser in my student town a few years later showed me what my hair could do and, apart from two pregnancies and a brief dabble with hair straighteners when I was 40, I had worn it curly ever since. It had been long, short and in between and while I had recently been debating with myself how long I could get away with home-dying it to cover the grey, and I was still searching for that elusive product that eliminates frizz and produces perfect sleek curls, I had made peace with my wild curliness.

In the first couple of months after my diagnosis, I cried the most tears over losing my hair, and that was before it happened. That felt rather shallow and I am almost embarrassed to admit it, but it is worth remembering that the thing that sparks our tears is not necessarily the thing we are really grieving about.

Whether we like it or not, appearance is very important to most people. It is how we present ourselves to the world and is closely connected to our identity. When we look in the mirror, we recognise what we see as who we are, even though we know that there is far more to us than what we look like. It is not surprising that the prospect of such a drastic change in appearance is upsetting but I think that my grief about losing my hair combined with all the other ways in which my sense of identity was being challenged by this experience of cancer, and my tears were for those deeper losses too.

I was intrigued about how other people coped with the loss of their hair. What did people use to cover their heads? Where do you get a wig and what type is best? What other options are there when you are convinced, like I am, that headscarves are a symbol of patriarchal oppression and to be avoided at all costs?

Cancer robs you of your normal choices about your appearance and forces you to make reluctant ones, and different people will do what works for them. Like so many other aspects of cancer that I was being initiated into, learning how to be bald felt like having to learn a new language, a bewildering challenge that I really did not want to have to undertake.

Some people are offered a 'cold cap' to wear while they are having chemotherapy which is designed to reduce hair loss, but I was told that it wouldn't work for the mix of drugs I was having and, besides, I hate being cold so hours with an ice pack on my head seemed like too much pain for too little gain.

I went to see Bianca, my hairdresser, a couple of weeks before my first treatment to get her to cut my long curly hair short in preparation. When I tried to explain what I wanted I burst into tears, which rather gave the game away that that was not what I wanted at all. Bianca got emotional too; several people in her family had died from cancer and for her a diagnosis felt little different to a death sentence. She gave me a big hug and refused to cut my hair short – 'why lose it before you have to?' – but she did give me a great haircut which saw me through the next few weeks.

I had been told at my first chemotherapy session that I would start to lose my hair in a couple of weeks and right on time, a fortnight later, as I was washing my hair in the shower it started to fall out, covering my hands and clogging up the plug hole. I was feeling elated after running five miles that morning so I wasn't that bothered – proof once again that running makes everything better – but perhaps it was more that I had become resigned to losing it.

After a few days of my hair coming out in handfuls, finding it in my food, and worrying what state it would be in for work on Monday, I went back to see Bianca and this time she cut it very short. I hoovered the house and put all my hair products at the back of the bathroom cabinet. I decided that Sinead O'Connor would be my role model and tried to feel positive about the next few months of being differently beautiful.

Early on, while I was commuting to work one day, I had seen a woman with a bald head waiting on the platform at Hammersmith tube station. I wasn't brave enough to go and talk to her, but her boldness and the fact that everyone just carried on around her made me wonder whether I could do that too.

On the way home after my second chemo treatment, just four days after Bianca had cut my hair for the second time, I stopped at an anonymous barber's on the walk back to the tube station and asked him to clipper my head because by now I had bald patches and tufty bits which looked ridiculous. I bit my lip and avoided making eye contact with myself in the mirror so that I didn't dissolve into tears. I wondered how many cancer patients walked out of Charing Cross Hospital and into his shop to do the same thing, but I was so emotional that I didn't trust myself to ask.

My cousin, Chris Wheelwright, lives in Texas and she had had treatment for breast cancer the year before me. She e-mailed me to say, 'When you become bald you are very definable as a woman who is going through cancer treatment; very few others choose this. With that identification comes a membership to an elite club of fantastic, strong, fighting, loving women. You will beat this. More good comes out of it all than bad. It will be over. Welcome to the club.'

After all my angst, Chris was right. The reality of being bald was not as bad as I had feared. Because I was having treatment in the summer, being bald turned into a pragmatic decision as much as an aesthetic one. Temperature dictated when I covered my head to protect it from the sun or the cold and I had a headband that made a very convenient beanie hat which I carried around with me, and which I could put on quickly without needing a mirror or much faffing around. I tried wearing headscarves a couple of times but felt profoundly uncomfortable wearing them. I didn't know how to tie them so they looked good, in spite of studying videos online.

I bought a wig early on that I ended up wearing only once. Jonny trains people in pioneering leadership and I went to his students' graduation in July. I wore the wig because it was his day and I didn't want to draw attention to myself but it left me feeling like I was in disguise, and not really myself, so I never wore it again. I ended up feeling that to be bald was to be true to who I was and what was happening to me at that moment.

It took courage at times to go into new places, or to meet people that had not seen me bald before, and there were a few work meetings where I felt a bit vulnerable and kept my beanie hat on rather than cope with what I thought other people's reactions might be. But I think it takes as much courage to wear a wig or a headscarf as it does to be bald, because we are having to look different to the norm, and different to what we would choose for ourselves if we still had control over that choice.

And of course there was plenty of over-analysing and angst on my part in the background behind that decision. Is being bald too 'in your face'? Does it look aggressive or make other people feel uncomfortable? Does it seem attention-seeking – 'look at me, I've got cancer!'? I realised that what mattered most was my motivation, not what other people thought about the choices that I made. And the people who were most important to me, my friends and family, were all very affirming; they couldn't all have been making it up to spare my feelings.

It was interesting to challenge the norms of feminine appearance, and to pay attention to how that made me feel. In the past, I had definitely felt more confident when I knew that I looked good whether that was through what I was wearing or my hair behaving for once, and that feels like a very insubstantial thing to base confidence on. I am getting older so my appearance is going to keep changing anyway, and I hoped that this experience would make it easier to age gracefully rather than trying to hold on to what I used to look like.

I changed my profile photos on social media fairly regularly during treatment to reflect my new baldness. I didn't want to pretend that I still had lots of hair, or to see that wild curliness as a standard that I had to reach again. Those current photos said, 'This is me and this is what I look like.' And I have to say that London was a great place to be a bald woman because no one batted an eyelid. That is partly because of our great British reserve, but partly because London is so diverse; we are used to people looking different.

I lost hair from all over my body of course, some of which was very welcome. You learn to appreciate the few perks of cancer treatment when they appear and several months of not having to shave my legs was a small bonus. My eyelashes disappeared which meant that if I was wearing eyeliner, the slightest hint of a tear would give me panda eyes as it all ran.

At school, I used to get called Denis Healey because I had a bushy monobrow to rival his. Over the years, I had divided it and tamed it into submission through plucking and threading, but my eyebrows were now a faint shadow of their former selves and I started colouring them in to lessen the scary cancer patient look. And strangely, I never went completely bald, as a sprinkling of hairs on my head stubbornly continued to grow in spite of the poison they were having to contend with.

When I was seven, my family moved house and I went to a new village junior school where everyone else had grown up together. I was invited to a little girl's birthday party and I wore my denim trousers that my mum had made for me – the closest I got to jeans at that age. I was growing out of them so she had sewn tartan patches on the knees and put a tartan band round the bottom of each leg to make them longer. I thought they were great until I turned up at the party and found that all the other little girls were in frilly pink dresses. The party girl came over to me and bent down to scrutinise the patches on my knees. 'Are they meant to be there?' she asked in a faux innocent voice while I shrivelled inside and wished I had stayed at home.

Small encounters like these can still have a disproportionate impact years after they have happened, even if you tell yourself that the opinion of a seven-year-old is not worth listening to. Ever since then I had tried to avoid the embarrassment of being the odd one out, particularly when it came to what I looked like. My few months of being bald help to lay to rest any remnants of lingering childhood shame at looking different to everyone else. It is strangely empowering to face your fears and find that that earns you respect rather than scorn. I would never have chosen to be bald, but for that short time it became who I was and I wore it well.

On Sorrow and Self-Pity

I felt sorrow creeping up on me as my fourth chemotherapy beckoned and with it the prospect of the long, deep dive into a muffled world. It is tempting to shrug it off – who wants to feel sad or be with someone who is sad? – but rather than resist it or fight it, I need to welcome sorrow as natural and needed in this season of my life.

My friend Becca, a youth worker who is studying for a PhD, had ME for two years. She tells me that you can't compare illnesses and hardships but it seems to me that ME is a particularly cruel and devastating illness, with no end in sight.

She wrote on her blog about the importance of accommodating grief, words that resonated with me even though my illness is very different to hers, 'Learning to accommodate ME is to accommodate grief. Everything that I realise I can't do, provides a new window of grief at this sadness that will not go away for as long as I am ill. Despite it being two years in, I am still grieving health and not living the life I'd hoped I would be. Sadness at not being able to do daily things that I so wish I could – cook a meal, walk home, see a friend, drive to the beach on my own, spend time with friends uninterrupted by tiredness and brain fog... Accommodating grief into my life feels like one of the most spiritually significant things I've had to do along the ME illness journey.'

Wanting to make the most of the days when I feel well, I have seen two animations at the cinema recently which explore emotions. *Song of the Sea* is the most beautiful and haunting film about a family coping with loss and grief. Ben and his silent sister Saoirse get caught up in a mission to save the spirit world that is in danger of being turned into stone by the owl witch Macha who captures negative emotions in glass jars in an effort to control the world around her. It is the type of film that stays with you long after you have seen it, and I would say it is the better film of the two.

Pixar's *Inside Out* also centres on emotions and the role they play in the life of a young girl called Riley whose family move to San Fransisco. It is less subtle than *Song of the Sea* but it had a profound effect on me.

Inside Riley's head are five emotions – Joy, Sadness, Fear, Anger and Disgust – who control how she responds to the world around her. Riley comes from a loving family and Joy is used to being in the driving seat, with the other emotions letting her take the lead. With the move to a new city, to a house that needs a lot of work, with no furniture due to a delayed removal van and a stressed dad, it is hard for Joy to stay in control but she tries none the less, especially as Riley's mum asks her to be happy to support her dad.

Whenever Sadness touches a memory, it turns blue which seems to threaten Riley's happy foundations, so Joy tries to contain Sadness by drawing a circle on the ground and insisting she stands in it. When Sadness is neglected she becomes whingey and difficult, refusing to walk by herself and needing to be dragged along by Joy who is trying to save the day.

When Joy and Sadness get locked out of the brain's command centre, Fear, Disgust and Anger take over, and Riley decides to run away and return to Minnesota. Joy and Sadness make it back, of course, but the resolution comes not by getting Joy back in the driving seat, but by letting Sadness take over. She holds the core memories that define who Riley is and they all turn blue, showing how the move has touched the very heart of her identity.

Riley finally tells her parents just how sad she is, and in her dad's embrace she is able to feel safe and start to smile again. Rather than being banished or controlled, Sadness needed to be at the forefront for a time and after she has been paid enough attention, Riley is able to move on to a more nuanced way of feeling and understanding emotions. Stories help us make sense of our lives and this rang so true for me; we need to sit with sorrow when she calls, until she has done her work.

But I have also been thinking a lot about self-pity – the toxic and self-indulgent wallowing in your woes that turns you in on yourself and distorts your perspective. It seems to me that there is a thin line between sorrow and self-pity, and while one leads back to life, the other only makes things worse.

On Tuesday I had three appointments lined up – with my chiropractor which is my treat to myself before chemotherapy, with my oncologist and then with the CT department for a scan of my abdomen, and none of them went well. Self-pity tapped me on the shoulder when I missed my chiropractor appointment because the District Line had long delays. She nudged me in the ribs a couple of hours later when the registrar told me that I need a port fitted because my veins are getting damaged. She breathed down my neck when the nurse couldn't cannulate me for a CT scan because those same veins are too inflamed in one arm and too fragile in the other, leaving bruises as a record of his attempts and leaving me afraid that chemo couldn't happen the next day.

It is so tempting to think 'poor me' but those things are inconvenient or random rather than part of a cosmic plot to make my life miserable. When I look at what so many people are going through around me and in the wider world, I have very little reason to feel that I am a victim.

Instead sorrow overwhelmed me when Jonny asked me later how my day had been and in talking about it I realised what was happening. A cancer diagnosis disrupts and destabilises your world, making you question what you thought you knew about it. A treatment plan offers a map to navigate this new territory and gives you a story to tell yourself – six treatments, surgery and I will be okay by Christmas. Then partway through things start to shift – the tumour isn't shrinking much, my liver is malfunctioning, my veins can't cope – and that map needs to be re-written.

I only have this one experience of cancer and while the medical team know what to do and what adjustments to make and it is just par for the course for them, I find it unsettling and scary. I need to grieve for the loss of control in my life, for the lack of ability to make plans and to stick to commitments. I need to grieve for my strong body that used to rise to any challenge and carry me through whatever was ahead. I need to grieve for the plans I want to make for next year and let them go, until I know what next year is going to look like. Being honest about that, having a good cry and a strong embrace from my husband helped so much and meant the run to chemo the next day was genuinely joyful and life-giving. Rosie, my chemo nurse and the queen of cannulas, put one in for the drugs and another for the CT scan and it was all fine.

Walter Brueggemann, the theologian, writes, 'Only grief leads to newness.' Whenever things change, we need to sit with sorrow and grieve for what is lost so that we don't get stuck in the old way of being and can embrace what lies ahead. Becca understands this and I think I am beginning to get it. So here's to spending time with sorrow when she needs attention. Here's to resisting self-pity when she breathes down my neck. And here's to the wisdom to know the difference.

7

More Chemotherapy

August and September

TO play any sport well, you need to train your mind as well as your body. As well as legs that can go the distance, you need to be able to deal with the angst and doubts that can creep in when the going gets tough. We say this to the people who join the beginners' group. Many of them, after the first session of mixed running and walking, wonder how they will ever manage to run continuously for 30 minutes or more. But somewhere over the next six weeks as they run more and walk less, they begin to trust what their body has done and expect that it can do more. Their internal 'I can't' turns into 'Wow – look! I can!' and a runner is born.

You need mental strength in a race of any length, but I had always found I most needed it in a marathon. The first half is fairly straightforward because I know that I have run this distance quicker many times, and usually the task is to stop myself going too fast. But around mile 16, I start to think, 'How can I carry on at this pace for a whole ten more miles?' The answer is not to worry about the next ten, but to run the mile you are in. Do one more mile. And at the end of that mile, just do one more. And so mile 16 soon becomes mile 18 which turns into mile 20 and so on. Inevitably I slow down towards the end but rather than being daunted by the next ten, I know I can do one more mile.

The fourth treatment out of six was looming. It was the equivalent of mile 17 in a marathon, and the pain was kicking in. The last treatment had been tough and I felt like I hadn't had much respite. Richard Tucson, an Eagles coach, had been having treatment for cancer a few weeks ahead of me. His advice was not to think of all the treatments at once. He sent me a message, 'It's like four reps in intervals. Always focus on the next one and worry about the others after the rest in between.'

So while my inner toddler had her arms folded and her bottom lip stuck out, while she was stamping her foot, red in the face and shouting 'but I don't WANT to go', my grown-up self had lined up her chemo run companions and was telling her that it will be all right; we can do this. One more mile.

This time Harry and Chris were running with me; Lucy was away on holiday. The previous day of hospital appointments had been stressful. I had been given a name for the state of my left arm, thrombophlebitis, and told that it was inflammation caused by the toxicity of the drugs.

It was still swollen and red, and I couldn't straighten it because the veins were like tight cords. I was going to have chemotherapy in my right arm today but would need to have a port fitted for the last two treatments, which would deliver the drugs straight into a deep vein in my chest rather than going through my arms.

All of this had caused me a lot of anxiety and I was catastrophising about whether my left arm would ever recover because no one seemed to know very much about it. The registrar had told me that it was the worst case of thrombophlebitis he had ever seen. My competitive side had immediately started to feel proud about that until I remembered exactly what I was supposedly 'winning' at, and I calmed down. I was also having a different drug, docetaxel, for the next three treatments which was all part of the original plan, and I had been warned that the side-effects could be worse.

This run was an oasis of calm in between hospital visits, an hour of conversation, exertion and normality that stopped me fixating on how difficult things were and brought me back to my true self. I had begun to feel that my body was letting me down with its misbehaving veins and malfunctioning liver; running reminded me of what it could still do and that I needed to nurture and be grateful for it rather than rail against it. Running to chemotherapy had started as an act of defiance, a refusal to surrender totally to the world of illness, but it had become an important component of my treatment, a place to process what was happening and to prepare for what was ahead. Once again it was a life-giving experience that left me light-hearted and ready for what was next. I slowed to a walk a couple of times to catch my breath, but having Harry and Chris there helped me keep going and we did the full seven miles of the river route.

After chemotherapy, I had to go and have a CT scan of my abdomen in preparation for the mastectomy and reconstruction I would have in the autumn. They had tried to do the scan the day before but had had trouble getting a cannula into my vein, and after three attempts and some impressive bruises I had stopped them so that they didn't totally ruin my veins for the next day. When I had talked to Dr Lewanski about running to chemo, he had commented that it could perhaps be beneficial because exercise increases the blood flow around your body and opens up your veins. It certainly seemed to have helped that day. The nurse, Rosie, had no trouble getting a cannula in my arm for chemo and then another one further up my arm for the dye they would inject into me for the CT scan, to show up where the blood vessels were. Maybe exercise was benefiting me in more ways than I first realised.

Cancer websites recommend exercise during treatment, but because they are giving general advice and most people are not very active, their recommendation is to walk for 30 minutes a day. When I had first read that I had thought perhaps that was all I would be able to do, because the treatment would be so harsh. I was so grateful to have had the encouragement of an oncologist who understood running, and why it was so important to me and I wondered how many active women curtailed their exercise unnecessarily when they got a cancer diagnosis because they thought they had to.

I had been reading up on exercise and breast cancer and was not surprised to find that it had many benefits. Exercise can boost the immune system and help to lessen the effects of 'chemo brain', the forgetfulness and fogginess caused by the drugs. It can reduce the risk of secondary cancers and improve people's quality of life. A few people had cautioned me that too much running would just wear me out, but the evidence suggests that regular exercise actually reduces fatigue rather than causing it and that was definitely my experience.

I got to know other women through social media who were staying active during their treatment. Liz O'Riordan was a triathlete and a breast surgeon with breast cancer. She had cycled up the Stelvio mountain pass in Italy a month before her diagnosis. She was cycling to some of her treatments, did parkrun regularly, swam, and even did her local sprint distance triathlon halfway through chemotherapy. I loved following her exploits on Twitter and reading her blog. I felt like I had found a kindred spirit even though we had never met.

I also connected with Alice-May Purkiss who had got into running just before she was diagnosed with breast cancer in her mid-20s. She had done a Cancer Research 10k the previous year and had immediately signed up for it again, obviously not realising that she would be in the middle of cancer treatment when it came round. Two days after her final chemotherapy she ran the race with a squad of friends and family, slowly but surely, finishing in tears but with a huge sense of achievement. She found running to be a safe space that gave her the freedom to feel everything she needed to, in a place that was just hers, something that I could really identify with.

Of course, people have different diagnoses and respond differently to treatment. I was fortunate that the cancer was superficial and had been caught relatively early. I went into my treatment feeling fit and well, so was starting from a positive place. Not everyone can sustain the same level of activity, nor should they feel like they have to try. Those of us going through cancer treatment need to listen to our bodies and do what we can cope with rather than setting ourselves unrealistic targets. No one should feel under pressure to exercise hard if that is not their thing. But I think more could be done to help people understand the many benefits of exercise, and to let active women and men know that a cancer diagnosis doesn't have to stop them doing the sport they love.

Two days after chemo, Jonny and I set off on holiday. Months previously, we had booked two weeks in a camper van in the Outer Hebrides. Jonny is a skilful photographer and was looking forward to capturing wild landscapes and moody sea scenes. I had been planning runs along deserted trails and beside the coast. But sense prevailed when cancer called. After my experience of swapping a graduation hall for A&E, I didn't want to be too far from medical help and I also didn't think I could cope with the discomfort of all that travel. I was often restless at night, but in a camper van there is nowhere else to go when you can't sleep which would mean both of us suffering.

We had switched the booking to a farm in Herefordshire for one week, followed by another at Pickwell Manor in Devon while Susie and Steve were away in France.

The Potting Shed was a quirky wooden lodge built at the bottom of the garden by the owners of the farmhouse. It had a tiny bedroom and a mezzanine space where Jonny slept so that I could toss and turn without disturbing him too much. Upstairs there was a balcony overlooking a field of cows where we ate our breakfast each morning. There were hammocks under the apple trees where I dozed during the day.

The effect of treatment was kicking in and this was an ideal place to endure it. Even though I had been through it several times already, the descent into feeling unwell was destabilising and distressing. There were the physical side-effects to contend with. My bones ached deep within my body and I could not get comfortable, whether sitting or lying down. This time my mouth was really tender and my saliva reflex triggered a strange intense pain every time I ate. My appetite and taste buds seemed to have disappeared, even though Jonny was cooking me wonderfully healthy food each day. It was hard to concentrate on anything and my energy was really low.

But the drugs also affected my perspective on the world and my sense of my place in it. Deep down, I wanted to take shelter, to hide away in a safe place, to make sure that all I needed was within reach. I was like a child who builds a den under the dining room table and hangs blankets over it to create soft walls that reduce the world to a manageable size, that create the illusion that this is all there is. I didn't have the energy to explore; I didn't want to make decisions; I wanted someone else to take care of life for me.

I retreated into childhood, took several steps back from the competent, taking-charge me. When I started to feel a bit better, Jonny and I went for a walk through some nearby fields. I felt incredibly anxious about where the paths were, and where we were allowed to go, not wanting to step out of line or be found in the wrong place. This was not me.

I found it hard to feel so vulnerable but I didn't feel I had any choice at the time, which was perhaps a good thing. I couldn't toughen up because I had nowhere to summon toughness from. I needed to let this be what it was, to remember that thankfully this was temporary for me, to be kind to myself, to accept all the help that was so generously offered. I needed to hold on to the promise that this, too, would pass and soon I would be running again.

It took Jonny and me a while to work out how to relate to each other in this unfamiliar space. Our relationship was shifting along with everything else. He asked me each day what I wanted to do, because he wanted to understand how I was feeling and to go at my pace. That felt such a pressure to me, like I was responsible for everything when I didn't have the mental energy to make decisions.

I felt guilty that he was having a crap holiday and it was all my fault. I went to bed at 9pm each day in a different room to him, while he stayed up by himself playing the guitar and drinking single malt. We had to feel our way towards each other. Twenty-eight years earlier we had promised to love each other in sickness and in health, and he was doing such a good job of that but I would much rather have been the carer than the cared for, the strong one instead of the sick one.

We hired a canoe and Jonny paddled me down the Wye River where we saw kingfishers darting across the water just in front of us. We went for a gentle stroll around a lake in Brecon, turning back all too soon because I couldn't manage the whole circuit. We spent several hours at Hereford Hospital when my arm swelled up again and managed to persuade a disinterested doctor to give me antibiotics. On our last day in Shenmore, I went out for a stumbly, hesitant run down the lane and across the field, the equivalent of the two laps of Ealing Common that I had done after each previous treatment to show myself that I could still do this.

In between Herefordshire and Devon, we stopped off in Bath to spend the weekend with our friends, Jon and Clare Birch. We had first got to know Jon when we had lived in Bath all those years before, and grew to love Clare when they got together. They are a warm and generous couple, who have a gift for welcoming people into their lives. Conversations at their house are always animated and opinionated; they are both champion ranters when they put their minds to it.

This was a safe space to be weak and ill. I didn't need to be interesting or entertaining; I could flop on their sofa and just be. Jon is a talented musician and designer who has suffered from anxiety over the years and doesn't travel far from his home. I sensed that he understood what I was feeling during chemotherapy perhaps more than anyone else, because he had had his own struggles with feeling insecure and afraid. Jon had shaved his head in solidarity with me, and while I was there he clippered my head to get rid of the few wispy bits of hair that still persisted in growing. Jonny took a photo of us together – two vulnerable baldies holding on to each other for dear life.

On the Saturday morning I persuaded Jonny to come and do Bath Skyline parkrun with me. I had done my first parkrun at the first Gunnersbury parkrun four years previously and in these days of running less, I was falling in love with it more. parkrun had been born over a decade previously in Bushy Park when Paul Sinton-Hewitt and his friends had started doing a timed 5k run every Saturday morning. It has become a global phenomenon with over 700 events happening each weekend around the world, with over two million registered parkrunners, and was still volunteer-run, free to enter and genuinely welcoming to all.

Even when you are visiting a new location as a tourist, there is a wonderful sense of familiarity about every parkrun – from the streams of runners making their way to the start, to the briefing about the route, from the sincere welcome to first timers and the heartfelt thanks to all the volunteers. I always think that these are my people; this is where I would start to make friends if I ever moved to a new town.

parkrun is where marathon finisher shirts line up next to not-been-worn-since-school plimsolls. It is where children take part alongside adults as soon as they feel ready to, and quickly find out they can beat a fair few of them. It is where dogs pull their owners round and athletic parents push children in buggies. Its 5k distance is long enough to present a real challenge to new runners, and difficult enough to keep even the most experienced coming back to chase down PBs. parkrun is for people who include it in their marathon training plan, and for those for whom it is their sole form of exercise. It is for people like me who that Saturday felt I couldn't go any further, but who a couple of days later find that actually they can. No one is too slow for parkrun. You can't get lost or left behind.

parkrun is the quiet witness to countless people turning their lives around, where good intentions to exercise first become a reality, where dreams of running a marathon 'someday' start to become a possibility. parkrun asks nothing of you, but gives you wonderful opportunities to contribute and engage, and a community to belong to if that is what you are looking for.

Bath Skyline parkrun is on the edge of the city in Combe Down, and is a beautiful route through woodland with stunning views. My run was slow and I had to walk up the steps near the start, while other runners bounded past me. Jonny had to wait for me a couple of times and I don't think I would have run all the way if he had not been next to me, but I loved it. It made me realise how much I had taken for granted being able to run long distances. I really appreciated the sense of achievement that finishing each parkrun gave me.

I usually described myself as a marathon runner to anyone that was interested. After my experience in Bath I changed my Twitter bio to 'parkrunner' instead, in keeping with my intention to be transparent about what was happening to me, but I was equally proud to number myself in that tribe.

Jonny drove us down to Devon and we settled into Pickwell Manor for the week. The weather was mixed but we spent time on the beach anyway, piling on the layers when it got cold and stripping them off when the sun appeared. I had favourite runs that I did every time I went down there, around Baggy Point or along the beach to Woolacombe, but each of them ended with a steep climb back up the hill to Pickwell. I did shorter versions instead, driving down to the car park next to the beach to start from there and driving home afterwards instead of clambering up the hill. It was an effort to run and the smallest incline seemed to defeat me.

I was still on antibiotics for my inflamed arm, and I was not sure whether my lack of energy was due to an infection or just the cumulative effect of all the drugs. Still it was good to be out in the open air and to be running, even if it was very slow.

Back in London, I started to gather my chemo runners for the next treatment. My sister Liz, who had run alongside her local river six weeks previously, had been in training so that she could come and run with me, and Mandy, not wanting to be left out, decided to come too. Chris was on holiday this time and Harry was up in Edinburgh performing at the festival, but Lucy was back and was up for another run.

The previous time I had seen Mandy, she had helped me sort through my wardrobe and get rid of all the clothes that I never wore. She arrived at my house that morning with some dresses that she had taken in for me, and some cushions that she had made out of old race t-shirts that were too tatty to wear but that I hadn't wanted to throw away. The cushion she made out of my Brighton Marathon finisher's shirt said, 'There will be days when you don't think you can run a marathon; there'll be a lifetime of knowing that you have.' I gave it pride of place on my settee.

In fact, instead of running to chemo number five, we were running to my port fitting which needed to happen first. Liz had never run seven miles before which I found strangely helpful. I was feeling a bit daunted by the distance but instead of worrying about myself I could worry about her. I was touched that while I had been enduring the treatment, she had been putting in the effort in training so she could come and be with me. I felt protective of her, but need not have worried because she managed it easily.

Now I was experiencing what it was like to be the slowest runner, to feel like you are holding people back, to know that I couldn't go much further, but also to realise that in this kind of run none of that mattered. It was about the experience of running, and the friendship of the people I was running with. In *Running with the Pack*, Mark Rowlands talks about the heartbeat of a run which is the essence of the run, what the run really is. The heartbeat of that run was solidarity – we are in this with you. They delivered me safely to the hospital where Jonny met us so he could accompany me through the procedure and take me home again.

The port was fitted at the top of the left-hand side of my chest under local anaesthetic. It was done beneath an x-ray machine so the surgeon could ensure that the tubes were going in the right place. A radiographer held my hand and stroked my arm all the way through, a kind gesture which I found reassuring. After a two-hour wait so they could check that I had coped with the operation okay, we were allowed to go home.

The next day I was back, this time travelling on the tube, to meet my friend Julie Johnson, who was going to sit through chemo with me. I was starting to feel demob-happy because, even though there were two periods of feeling awful to go, it felt like the end was in sight. I was upbeat as the nurse attached a tube to my new port and the docetaxel started to drip into my body, and Julie was a great companion to do it with, feeding me grapes and keeping me distracted.

We had met when we both worked for the same charity, and Julie had written a drugs education video for small children that I had produced. We had acted as peer mentors to each other when we both worked as consultants, meeting up to talk about how our work was going and then putting the world to rights over cocktails and good food. To be honest there had probably been more of an emphasis on the food and cocktails than the actual mentoring bit, but ours was an energising friendship that I really valued and I was grateful that Julie was here to share this experience with me.

The descent into the fog of chemo was now tediously familiar, and again it seemed to hit me harder still. The three-week cycle of chemo gives your body a chance to recover in between, but each time I had not quite got back to my level of well-being at the start, and I was gradually getting weaker overall.

I was fit and well when I had the first treatment; now my default setting was to feel vulnerable, unsure and disabled. My mouth was even more tender and I couldn't cope with any amount of chilli in my food. My fingernails had discoloured as if there were blood blisters behind them, and my fingertips were numb and swollen. The beds of my fingernails were incredibly sore and I had to be careful when I put my hand in my bag or my pocket in case I accidentally jarred them against something, which set the nerves jangling.

My feet were suffering too, painful and covered in blisters, and the only shoes that were comfortable were my trainers. I had to write the final assignment for my masters, and somehow cobbled together enough words on the theme to hit the target. I handed it in, knowing that it was the worst piece of academic work I had ever written but really not caring because I had nothing else to offer.

Ten days after chemo number five, I did my slow two laps of the common, proof that I was coming back to life. Shortly afterwards it was time to go back to work and I felt really ambivalent about it. The decision to keep working during chemotherapy, to do one week in three, had been instinctive when I found out I had cancer. I felt responsible at work and I didn't want to duck out of that, nor did I know how the treatment was going to affect me and I didn't want to anticipate the worst and give up too soon.

It had been good to stay connected and to have a reason to be focused outwards, and my workplace and work colleagues had been incredibly supportive. Cancer was cocooning me from the outside world in many ways. People were protecting me, doing things for me, lessening the stress of everyday life, and I was very grateful for that, but going to work stopped me being too self-centred and extended the boundaries of what I thought I could do; it stopped my world getting too small. Without it, I could easily have got isolated and insular. I was aware that I was very privileged in so many ways. Some people have no choice about whether they work or not, and many have caring responsibilities that only intensify when they are ill.

But inevitably work brought its own stress and added pressure and I didn't feel like I was doing it very well at all. The pattern I had chosen meant that I spent the weeks when I felt most well and had most energy in the office, rather than simply enjoying a return to something like normality, but I wasn't able to do much outside of work because it exhausted me.

From time to time I asked myself whether it was the right decision to keep working, but I came to the conclusion that that was the wrong question. There is no right answer to the challenge of how to deal with cancer. So much is unknown and we just have to make the best decisions we can with the information we have, and then adapt as things become clearer, which seemed to me a good way of dealing with life in general. There were many things

I hoped I could leave behind in this season, and the need to always get things right was one of them.

Time to arrange my final run to chemotherapy. Lucy, Liz, Mandy and Harry were signed up and Neil, another Eagle, was going to join us. I had met Neil on his first club run a couple of years earlier when I had been the tail runner, there to go at the pace of the slowest runner so that no one got left behind. He had just moved to Ealing and hadn't done much running recently so we stuck together and chatted as we ran.

Neil had been through his own experience of cancer so he was one of the first people in the club that I told when I got my diagnosis. We had met up for coffee several times over the previous few weeks, and it had been really helpful to talk to someone who had experienced some of what I was going through. And then Joel rang me to say that he was going to come too. He was not a regular runner although he did play football once a week, and I was delighted that both my boys were going to be with me.

On the day, things did not quite go to plan. Liz lives in Harpenden and she got held up in traffic on the M1 as she drove down to Ealing. Joel texted to say that he had left the house with just his Oyster card and no money, and had discovered at London Bridge that he didn't have enough credit to get all the way to our house. He had rung Kat, who was on maternity leave and just days away from her due date, but she was still asleep so he wasn't sure if he would be able to make it.

I knew I would be slower still this time so didn't want to leave the house too late, and in the end Mandy, Harry and I set off to meet Lucy and Neil in the park before Liz or Joel had arrived. On the way, I got another text from Joel to say that Kat had rescued him with some money and he would get a train to Kew Bridge. As we ran along the road to the station, I could see him waiting at the end for us and we set off along the familiar river route for the final time.

This run was the antithesis of what I was running to. It was light-hearted, celebratory, and felt really significant. With the help of my friends and family, I had run to all my chemo treatments along the river even though my body and spirit were battered and bruised, my arm was deformed and my feet were blistered. I felt a real sense of achievement.

The slogan of Right to Movement, the running community that organise the Palestine Marathon, is 'we run to tell a different story'. Running to my chemotherapy appointments had enabled me to tell a different story about my treatment. It was a story about agency and determination, choosing to get to hospital on my own feet rather than completely succumbing to the passivity that accompanies being a patient. It was a story about solidarity, about people entering the cancer space I was forced to inhabit and being present with me. It was a story about joy, the simple, liberating, heartfelt delight of feet beating out a rhythm on the ground. It was a story about identity, holding on to who I was and what was important to me when I felt that I was losing everything.

Of course, it was also a story about anxiety and debilitation, sorrow and loss – those things were inescapable – but rather than them being the dominant themes that obscured everything else, they were sub-plots in a wider, richer narrative.

Kat met us at Charing Cross Hospital. Having been dragged out of bed by Joel, she thought she might as well come and say hi. Liz had been in touch en route to say that she had finally made it to Ealing and was going to run the route on her own. She arrived at the hospital half an hour after us and we all had lunch together at the Maggie's Centre, filling their courtyard with happy, sweaty runners. Harry stayed with me for my final dose of drugs and I went home thankful that this part of the treatment was over, and at the same time dreading the final dip to come.

My mum had taken very seriously my advice to her after my dad died, to go out walking so that she got her fitness back after months of hardly leaving the house. She bought the same type of fitness tracker as her brother and his wife, John and Meg, and connected to them online, so they could monitor each other's progress and get highly competitive. Each time she'd been to stay with me over the last few months, we had to make sure she did her steps each day, particularly if there was a chance that John or Meg might beat her total. Although she'd never been a runner, I think that becoming a dedicated walker gave her an insight into my addiction to running because it gave her so many of the same benefits.

Not wanting to be left out of marking the end of my treatment, she organised a walk for that evening with John and Meg, and my sister Susie and her family. She made everyone signs to wear on their backs which said 'Running with Jen' and they wore crazy pink wigs, sunglasses, umbrellas and hats. They walked along the river in Ely, naturally, and through the local nature reserve, getting smiles and thumbs up from people they met and offers of donations once people found out what it was all about.

There was an e-mail waiting for me when I arrived home from the hospital with photos attached which made me smile. I sang the Sister Sledge song to myself; all my sisters had made the effort that day to be with me. Susie, the youngest in our family, is an assistant head teacher and it had been difficult for her to come and visit me because of work pressures and illness but she had kept in touch regularly over the last few months and her support was no less precious because it was from a distance.

On Sunday we woke up to find an invitation from Joel to join a new group on our phones called Baby Time! along with Kat's family. Kat had been woken up by contractions at three that morning, her due date, and her waters had broken at six. They headed into the hospital soon after and managed to keep us updated, while we all sent messages of encouragement. Kat's family were all saying how typical it was that she was going to have her baby bang on time.

And at 2.30pm that day, Florence Elizabeth Baker was born. Jonny and I couldn't keep away. He drove me over to Lewisham Hospital and we met our granddaughter that afternoon. The chemo fog was descending, my bones ached and my progress through the hospital corridors was painfully slow but how wonderful to look into her little face, to hug Joel and Kat and to celebrate this new life. It brought back memories of when Joel was born and Jonny and I had been in their place, overwhelmed with the responsibility of caring for a new baby, in awe of this little person that we had played a part in creating and full of optimism and hope for the future. Flo's birth brought a promise of life returning, of happy days ahead, of loving and being loved.

When you are busy with work and the stresses and demands of everyday life, the thought of a day with nothing to do seems so attractive. When you are in those kind of empty, undemanding days, it is very different. I felt I ought to be doing something meaningful with all this free time, but a thick blanket of chemo haze muffled any remnants of energy or enthusiasm and I just got through the next week as best I could. I had felt so elated after my final run to Charing Cross and was excited about Flo being born, but neither of those things could penetrate far into the weariness that had descended into my body, mind and soul. I found it hard to be a weaker version of myself. I felt tender somehow, as if I was walking around with an outer layer of myself peeled away.

I was reading *Daring Greatly* by Brené Brown where she talks about the importance of vulnerability for a wholehearted life, but even she recognises that it is unhealthy to be vulnerable with everyone all the time, that there is a time and a place for it; I felt that I had little choice. I had always enjoyed getting things done and doing them well, but I didn't feel that I was doing anything very well at all – work, running, friends, study, making plans. And I knew that that was how it had to be.

It wasn't that I was expecting too much of myself, more that I was missing out on something that is essential to everyone's well-being – a sense of competence and achievement. I think that is the way we are made, that we have gifts and talents that we need to use to feel fully human, and it is hard if our usual outlets for doing what we love are denied to us. I was struggling but I found myself saying, 'This is not how it will end.' How I feel today is not how this will end. The pain in my feet and my fingers is not how this will end. The lack of energy I have is not how this will end. My feelings of despair and sorrow are not how this will end.

And then ten days after the final treatment, I did a slow two laps of the common and the world seemed full of possibility again! Getting back outside in my trainers, even when the run was hesitant and included some walking, was the sign that my strength was returning. Finally, I could allow myself to feel a sense of relief that the chemotherapy was over.

The following Saturday, I joined Tracey Melville at her 100th parkrun. It was also the anniversary of her being told that her lymphoma was in remission and she had invited lots of friends to come and celebrate with her. She looked really well and was so happy to be running. I started out really pleased for her, but halfway round I saw Richard Tucson, who had just finished his cancer treatment, and stopped to give him a hug.

As I set off again, tears rolled down my cheeks and I cried as I ran round the rest of the route. I so desperately wanted to be where they were, at the end of all my treatment, beginning to get back to normal, looking back at cancer as something in the past. I knew that I was projecting my expectations on to them; I had no idea if that is what they were feeling or if I would feel like that once the treatment was over. But I was suddenly aware of what a heavy burden cancer was to carry and how I didn't want to have to carry it any more.

Jonny had gone on ahead of me and was waiting as I crossed the line and entered the finishers' funnel. I sobbed on his shoulder for several minutes, causing havoc with the timing tokens because I should have kept moving, but the woman in charge managed to sort it all out. Running seemed to be a place where I could feel everything I needed to, where I was able to access what was going on in my soul. It was a cathartic and emotional parkrun, and probably just what I needed.

That afternoon, Mandy and I got the train to Bath to stay the night with Jon and Clare. I had had to pull out of the Bath Two Tunnels Marathon, but Mandy had been training hard for it over the last few months and I wanted to be there to cheer her on. The race follows some of the Two Tunnels Greenway, a path along the route of the old Somerset and Dorset railway line. Each lap of the two-lap marathon goes through two railway tunnels, one 400m long and one just over a kilometre long, so it can call itself the UK race with the longest distance run underground.

Jon and Clare lived really close to the start so we waved Mandy off, wandered back to their house for coffee, and then went out again to stand by the route and wave as she went past for the second time. We were there to cheer her over the finishing line in a time of 5 hours and 2 minutes, just beating my first marathon time. She finished with a sprint and huge smile on her face; I was immensely proud of her.

My 18-week chemo plan was coming to an end, rather appropriately, with a race, the Ealing Half-Marathon. After my fourth treatment, which was my first dose of the deadly docetaxel, I had had to admit to myself that getting back up to running ten miles in between treatments in the hope that I could do a half-marathon just wasn't going to happen. It hadn't been too hard to let go of because I felt so weak and I knew that running that distance was completely beyond me.

But I had signed up to be a volunteer at EHM instead. I chose to be a road marshal at mile 12 so I could cheer people on in the final stage of their race. For the first hour and a half of being on duty there was not much to do; I chatted to the other marshals and gave directions to cars that needed to negotiate the road closures. Then came the lead bike and after him, the first runner making it look incredibly easy. There was another pause of several minutes, then a trickle of more runners that gradually turned into a flood for the next couple of hours, filling the road with bodies, effort and determination.

We clapped and cheered, shouting out encouragement: just one more mile to go; you've got this; you're looking strong; you can do it. So many familiar faces in the throng, each person running their own race, conquering doubts, discovering what they could achieve. The flood gradually slowed to a trickle again, and by now there was more pain on people's faces as they approached the end of their race. We cheered all the more, willing people on to the finishing line. Then came the tail-runner, the tail car, the traffic guys moving the 'road closed' signs out of the way and it was all over. I had sore hands and a croaky voice from cheering, but also a deep sense of joy.

If there was some way of measuring the well-being in a community then it would have rocketed that day, from people achieving PBs or doing their first half-marathon, from family and friends supporting and cheering people on, from volunteers making it all run smoothly, from children doing the mini mile and getting the running bug, from people giving and receiving, supporting and encouraging.

Someone reminded me of the poem in Ecclesiastes that begins, 'There is a time for everything and a season for every activity under the heavens.' I was tired of treatment and the limitations it placed on me. It felt like it had been dragging on for months but there was still a long way to go. What sort of time was I in at the moment? What was required of me?

A time to be and to endure;
A time to stay connected and to receive the love of family and friends;
A time to be kind to myself and allow myself to be cared for;
A time to choose gratitude and to find pleasure in small things;
A time to be open to new things and new friendships;
A time to heal and to choose life, to reflect and grow;
A time when joy and sorrow are close companions;
And a time that will come to an end.

Lizzy Hawker: Runner

At the risk of sounding obsessed, while I have been running less, I have been reading more about running. Lizzy Hawker is the most incredible athlete who is hardly known outside the world of ultrarunning. She has competed in the Ultra Trail du Mont Blanc six times, a race of over 150km up, down and around Mont Blanc, winning it five times and coming second once. She held the world record for distance covered in 24 hours in 2011, and won gold at the 100km world championships in 2006.

Her book *Runner* tells the story of these runs, as well as the incredible runs she has done from Everest Base Camp to Kathmandu. It is a fascinating insight into her love of mountains, running and solitude and the strength of character that enables her to keep on running.

I expected to be inspired by her story, to feel envious of the running she's done, to have my dream of doing an ultra 'one day' renewed, but I was not expecting it to be relevant to where I am at the moment. The third section of the book is about the injuries that she has been wrestling with more recently – six stress fractures in her legs, one after the other, over the course of two years. Just as she recovers from one and plans her next race, she gets another and is forced to rest.

She writes about the challenge this is to her sense of identity, the need to yield to the ways things are rather than resisting, and the importance of dancing on the right side of the line between strength and vulnerability. Here are some of her words that particularly resonated with me; where she writes about injury, I related it to illness:

'Injury is a hard master, a hard teacher. One that we don't always like to listen to. And yet in the dark places it can take us there is also a wonderful depth of opportunity. The delicate dance between injury and health gives us a space rich in opportunity to learn and to change. Life is shaped by our attitude, by our perception of what it is that is happening, and that is our choice. That is always our choice.'

You can tell that she would love to finish the book with a happy ending, with another ultrarun even if she didn't win it. She says, 'I struggle over the prospect of trying to finish *Runner* with an unfinished story of injury: "Wouldn't the message be stronger that I can go through a tough time and come out the other side, in whatever way that turns out to be?" You tell me bluntly, "But the other side is the dealing with the tough time, not the eventual phoenix rising from the flames." Yes, this is the real story, the tough time. Life is not a race, there is no finish line, there is no ending, happy or unhappy. All that we have is the journey that we are making and the attitude with which we make it. There is a powerful opportunity in this chaos if I just have the courage to rest in its uncertainty.'

I am not claiming that I am like Lizzy Hawker in any way other than sharing that love of running, but her words have made me think and helped me see again the opportunity in this season of my life to learn and grow. You don't become a saint when you have cancer; well, I haven't. All my insecurities and weaknesses are still present, and often magnified by the things I am facing. I think many of us, when life is going well, look at the tough times that other people are going through and wonder how we would cope if we had to face the same.

This is the year I have had to discover how I cope with having cancer, but I don't think I will fully know the answer to that until it is all over one way or another. None of us would choose something like this and I don't want to romanticise it in any way at all because it is horrible – not only for me but those who love me, but it has made me appreciate things that I have taken for granted for far too long – my family, my friends, my faith, my freedom.

Becoming a Grandma

Here is another golden moment in this strange season of my life. On Sunday, my wonderful daughter-in-law Kat gave birth to Florence Elizabeth and our whole family was transformed. The year before I had spoken at Joel and Kat's wedding and described it as a shift in the cosmos, a moment that changed all of us who were there. And this is another.

With Flo's arrival, everyone has a new name – mum, dad, uncle, great-grandma – and a new person to get to know. There is something very mysterious about newborn babies and their hidden internal lives. We might look for family likenesses but we have to wait for her true self to be revealed. Her future is full of potential and possibilities and we watch to see how it will unfold and who she will become. But instantly our hearts have expanded to embrace this new life, she's on my mind all of the time and I have bound my life to hers without question.

We went to meet Flo a few hours after she was born and even through the fog of chemo, there is something profoundly moving about seeing your boy hold his baby girl. I can still remember the elation and bewilderment of those first days after giving birth to Joel, the sense of wonder and amazement at this new life, alongside feeling totally overwhelmed by the responsibility of caring for him.

Now Joel and Kat need to find their way through these early days and weeks of being parents and I have no doubt that they will do it brilliantly, with grace and love and laughter. For them too there is a becoming, a growing into relationship and responsibility, a transition into parenthood.

Because although Flo's birth has changed us all, we need to grow into those new relationships and fully inhabit them. In one sense I became a grandma automatically at that moment of her birth, but in another it is the invitation of a lifetime and not something to take for granted. I don't feel old enough of course, but I have been thinking about what kind of grandma I hope to be. I want to be involved in her life so that I get to know Flo and she gets to know me. I want to be respectful and affirming of Joel and Kat as her mum and dad, and the choices they make about how they bring her up.

Flo has been born into a large extended family and a wide circle of friends and I want to play my unique part in that, contributing what I can to enrich her life, not least alongside my fellow grandparents, Jonny, Jan and Greg. I am looking forward to learning from her, and for my life to be enriched by the experiences we share together. And while I need to be guided by Joel and Kat and Flo herself, I want to be someone who opens up possibilities for her and helps her navigate the pink restrictions that are so often placed on girls, so that she thrives and blossoms and becomes the mighty girl that she was born to be.

8

Surgery

October to December

I WOULD never describe cancer as a gift, but there are gifts and opportunities to be found in its destructive wake. The marathon of chemotherapy had been a hard slog, but taking stock after it was over I realised how much I had enjoyed spending more time with my family, in deepening old friendships and forging new ones.

I loved having time to reflect and to write and I missed that when I wasn't able to do it as much in the weeks when work took over. I had been very touched and uplifted with the love and support that people had shown me in different ways, whether up close or at a distance. I had learned a lot about myself and had seen both the best and worst bits of my character up close. It is interesting to find out how much you can endure, and sobering to realise that you can still be a bitch even when you have cancer.

My approach had been to stay with one stage of my treatment at a time. There is a thin line between being prepared for what is next, and overthinking and catastrophising about what lies ahead. Chemo had filled my horizon for several months but now it was time for the next item on the cancer treatment list – surgery. I had known since May that I would need a full mastectomy because the cancer was multi-focal; as well as the large tumour I had found there was at least one other small tumour in the same breast. I would also have axillary clearance, the removal of all the lymph nodes under that arm, because there was cancer in at least one of them.

Over the previous few months I'd had several appointments with Jude Hunter, the plastic surgeon who would reconstruct my breast after Ms Shah had cut out the cancer. She had explained the various options in great detail to me – to simply have the breast and nipple removed, to have it reconstructed with an implant or to use my own body tissue to create a new 'breast'. In addition I could choose to have the reconstruction done at the same time as the mastectomy or wait to have further surgery later.

There had been some discussion about whether I had enough spare flesh to fill a new boob, but the slightly squidgy mummy tummy bequeathed me by my boys was deemed to be enough. What a bizarre set of choices to have to make, when actually I didn't want to have any of those done.

Years before I had resolved not to play the 'fight ageing' game that the beauty industry seduces women into and had decided that I would never have plastic surgery no matter how saggy or wrinkly I got. Now I found that decision had been taken out of my hands, although I did get to choose what type to go for. Implants would probably need to be replaced every ten years or so, and could be problematic combined with the radiotherapy that I would need.

Using my own tissue also carried risks but I wanted to minimise the need for any future surgery and liked the fact that my new 'breast' would be soft and warm, feeling more natural. I chose to have a DIEP reconstruction that would use skin and fat from my abdomen, leaving the muscles underneath intact. A blood vessel from the abdominal tissue would be reattached to one in my chest, keeping the tissue alive in its new location.

It was strange to think that these were the last few days with my right breast. I was grateful that I had been able to breastfeed my boys, for the sexual pleasure it had given to Jonny and me, that it had been an important part of my femininity. I was mindful of the thousands of miles of running it had done with me, jiggling around encased in a sweaty sports bra, and of the amount of prodding and poking it had had to endure over the last few months of scans and biopsies and check-ups. I was apprehensive about losing my breast but I hoped that like losing my hair, like the chemotherapy itself, the thought of it beforehand would be worse than the reality.

I spent the week before my surgery finishing off things at work, and handing over my responsibilities for the next few weeks; I was expecting to be back at work just before Christmas. I made the most of feeling well and had friends round for supper, went out for dinner with Jonny and spent some time with Florence. I bought pyjamas for hospital and front-fastening sports bras for afterwards.

The night before the operation I joined the Eagles club run, a bittersweet four miles through city streets and parks, running with friends, very aware that this would be my last run for at least six weeks. Although I had only done one of the four stages of treatment, I was convinced that chemo was the worst and that it would be plain sailing from here. I was more concerned about how I would cope without running than about the surgery. I thought I was ready.

Jonny went with me to Charing Cross Hospital early the next morning. We joined a waiting room full of apprehensive people where hardly anyone spoke. I had no words left, just a mute acceptance that I had to do this next stage. We were called through and I got changed into a hospital gown. Jude went through the consent forms that I had to sign and drew on my body with black marker pen, a big arrow pointing to my right breast, a circle around the nipple and lines across my abdomen indicating where they would make the incisions. Jonny was standing opposite me, watching the abstract conversations of the last few months being inscribed on my body in front of his eyes.

Then it was time for a hug goodbye, a walk to theatre, introductions to the anaesthetists and welcome oblivion. For the next nine hours, I was the still centre of a hive of activity. A team of people worked on and around me, removing this threat to my life, putting my relationship to cancer into the past tense, from 'I have...' to 'I had...', reshaping my body while I slept, unknowing.

Early that evening, I came round in the recovery room thinking that my heels were really painful and trying to work out why that was. I was lying under a heated blanket, drifting in and out of consciousness. Every hour, someone came to check the blood supply to the reconstruction using a Doppler machine, pressing the end of its wand to a stitch on my new breast that showed where the blood vessel was, until the pulse of a heartbeat filled the room. All I could do was sip water through a straw then go back to sleep, coming round again to the sound of my heart steadily doing its work, and with it the reassurance that the surgery had been successful. All through the night nurses came and went, watching over me while I slept fitfully, my head full of weird dreams.

The next morning I could assess the aftermath of the surgery. The black lines that Jude had drawn the previous day were now dark red gashes held together with glue. An impressive wound ran across my abdomen, a small one surrounded my belly button and another circled my strangely smooth, nipple-less right breast. I had four drains poking out of my sides, one on the left and three on the right, leaking bloody fluid into large plastic bottles. Compression sleeves on my lower legs inflated regularly with air, squeezing my calves tight and releasing them again. Of course there was nothing wrong with my heels at all.

The long hours of anaesthetic the previous day had left me feeling groggy and sick. I was completely helpless, dependent on other people to do everything for me. The regular checks on the blood supply to the reconstruction continued; each time the sound of the heartbeat brought a sense of relief that it had worked. Jude and her team did the ward round and said they were really pleased with how the operation had gone. It was good to have their reassurance as I just didn't know what to think about it. The procedure had happened exactly as they had described it to me, but it is one thing to see a diagram of what will happen and a very different experience to have those lines etched into your body with a scalpel.

That afternoon, the nurses wanted me to get out of bed and sit in a chair. They raised the head of my bed to a more upright position but my blood pressure was low and I nearly fainted; the chair was abandoned and I was allowed to sleep some more. I was struck by how weak I was if sitting in a chair was too much of a physical challenge for my body to cope with. Two days before I was running; now I couldn't even sit up. I had no reserves of energy left or even the desire to make myself do it. I was quite happy to be left alone to sleep.

I managed to sit in a chair the next day, but the goals kept coming. They wanted to remove my catheter and for me to walk to the toilet, carrying my drains in plastic bags. They wanted me to have a shower by myself. They wanted me to go for a walk round the ward so that I got some exercise. They wanted me to do a poo. Each of these seemed an overwhelming and impossible challenge at first and I resisted them. The nurses calmly insisted however and of course I achieved them one by one, slowly getting a little of my strength and dignity back.

Walking was particularly slow and tortured. The wound on my abdomen was so tight that I couldn't stand up straight, and I had to carry my drains everywhere I went. I hobbled slowly, clutching my plastic bags filled with bloody bottles, bent over like a cartoon drawing of a little old lady. I was scared that my wound would burst if I tried to stand up any straighter. Jude assured me that would not happen and I told myself to stop being so over-dramatic. Various members of my family came to visit over the next few days. Joel and Kat sneaked Flo in and held her up so that I could stroke her face.

Five days after the surgery I was allowed to go home with just one drain left. I took shelter in our spare room because it was next to the bathroom. It had been Harry's bedroom when he was a child and it still had luminous stars, planets and sheep over the walls and ceiling. I had to sleep on my back with the drain down the right side of the bed, and pillows under my shoulders and knees to keep my back in a curve because I couldn't lie flat. The next morning I was hit by a deep grief at the loss of my strong body. In hospital I had just been in survival mode, doing what the nurses told me with little space to reflect. Going home highlighted the difference between what I had been like last time I was here and how I was now, and made me think, 'What the fuck just happened?' To be honest, I think this was when I really had to face the fact that I had cancer. The tumour had not made me feel ill even though it had been growing in my body for months. My knowledge of cancer was intellectual rather than physical; I didn't *feel* like anything needed to be fixed.

All the treatment, however, was an assault on my body and surgery in particular felt brutal and disproportionate. I looked at my reconstructed breast and my slashed torso and thought, 'Was that really necessary?' Of course it was, but there had been a disconnect between what I knew in my head and what I felt in my body. Surgery highlighted that divide and forced me to confront it, giving me a very physical understanding of what having cancer meant. I wept and wept for the strong body that I had lost. I knew that I needed to accept this weaker, rearranged version of myself but it was hard.

The reconstruction looked peculiar and I was anxious about whether it had been successful. My hunched-over posture and tentative steps constantly reminded me of what had just happened. So much of me seemed to have been destroyed – my appearance, my strength, my mobility, my confidence. Was there anything left? How wrong I had been about the impact surgery would have on me.

There is an interconnectedness between body, mind and spirit. We use those words to describe different aspects of ourselves as if they were distinct and separate elements, but they are not. A healthy body, mind and spirit is an integrated whole, even if at times they get out of synch with each other as I had just experienced. Those words are different names for the same entity which is me. I am flesh and blood, awareness and memories, energy and mystery. What happens to my body has an impact on my mind and touches my spirit. To have the surface of your body cut by a knife is a violation, even if it is necessary, even if you submit to it willingly, even if it is done skilfully. The impact of surgery goes deep and the wounds it leaves are many.

I felt better after that storm of weeping, and there were many tears that followed. I found it difficult to come to terms with the reconstruction; I still couldn't think of it as my breast. The skin on it was broken and oozing, and I had to make several visits to the plastic surgery clinic at the hospital to get the dressing changed, and to have fluid drained. My right arm was tender and sensitive because the nerves had been affected when the lymph nodes were removed, a normal consequence of that kind of surgery, but another source of awkwardness and pain.

I worried that I had made the wrong decision about what surgery to have; perhaps I should have had an implant instead? I worried that the reconstruction felt lumpy and wondered if that meant it had not been successful. I talked to Jude about it when I saw her, and the dressing clinic nurses who dealt with this kind of thing every day, but I found it hard to trust their reassurances and wondered what they weren't saying to me.

I wished I had asked more questions and done more research before the operation. And I realised that all of this was part of the grieving process for what I had lost. I was in the 'death' part of the life-death-life cycle that is the recurring shape to all of our lives, and there was no way to avoid it; I needed to go through it. I reminded myself of what I had said earlier – there is no 'right' way to do this. You make the best decision you can with the information you have at the time. Whatever I had chosen would have been difficult to come to terms with; that is the very nature of what I was dealing with.

Over the next few days and weeks I gradually got stronger and as my body healed, my heart and soul slowly had time to catch up. I listened to Lemn Sissay on Radio 4's *Desert Island Discs* programme one day and found a deep resonance with what he said. A poet, writer and playwright who had recently been elected as chancellor of Manchester University, Lemn was fostered until he was 12 by a very religious family against his birth mother's wishes. He was a very happy child who loved his foster family. 'I thought everyone in the world smiled. I didn't realise that it was me smiling at the world, smiling back at me,' he says.

But when he was 12, on the verge of adolescence, his foster family put him into care and said that they would never write to him or contact him again. He lived in a succession of children's homes for the next five years, forced to form new relationships each time he was moved. Poetry enabled him to articulate and process what had happened to him and he had been able to forgive his foster family for what they did.

Towards the end of the programme, Kirsty Young asked him whether he was now at peace with his past and content with who he is. He said, 'The most important lesson I learned was to let go of anyone who doesn't want to talk to me, and to accept anybody who does, not to hold on to this narrative and not to hug the bruise. I am not defined by my scars, but by the incredible ability to heal. You have to live in the present, not in the past or in the future.'

Two weeks on, I was marvelling at my body's incredible ability to heal. Already the skin on my abdomen had knitted together and the angry red wound was becoming a fainter pink scar. Already I was walking further and straighter than in those first few days at home. I was faithfully doing my arm exercises, and already I could stretch my right arm further up the wall. I was starting to come to terms with the changes in my body and what would be my new normal. I was gradually getting less grumpy and reclusive, and more inclined to face the world.

There was a long way to go, of course. A week after the operation, Jonny had driven me to Pen Ponds in the middle of Richmond Park. I was desperate to get out of the house and be properly outdoors. I very slowly walked from the car park to the water's edge and back, a couple of hundred metres at most, wondering if I was going to make it, all the while thinking that the last time I had been there was when I was passing through on a long run to my friend Julia's house in Streatham Hill. It was impossible not to be aware of those contrasts but I was trying to observe them with interest, rather than them becoming a comparison heavy with regret. There is no going back once you have had cancer. It is not helpful to see your former achievements as a standard you have to regain. I really hoped that I would get back into running, and I hoped that would include long distances but that needed to be something that comes out of a future passion rather than trying to relive what I did in the past.

I didn't want to be defined by my scars either but I needed to accept that I was now scarred by the experiences of this year. My healed body and soul would be different to the original, but that would be okay. Lowell Sheppard, a Canadian friend, wrote to me around that time.

I had worked with him when I first moved to London and shortly afterwards, he and his wife Kande had gone to live in Japan, responding to a deep sense of calling on their lives. Kande had been born and grew up in Japan so was at home with the language and the people. Lowell didn't speak a word of Japanese and didn't have a job when they first moved there, but he had approached the move with a sense of adventure and had discovered a way to thrive in such a different culture. Sport had played an important part in that. He was a keen cyclist and had written a book about a cycling trip he had done around the coast, chasing the cherry blossom as it opened in the spring and attending the ceremonies that are held to celebrate its arrival.

Lowell wrote to me about the pottery town that he and Kande live in, 'We have potters all around us, and people come from all over the world to learn pottery from these dedicated artists. The most beautiful pieces are the ones that appear broken. I enquired about these some time ago and they said the broken objects are of more value than the pristine and new ones. They even have a technique called Kintsugi, which is the art of repairing broken pottery with lacquer mixed with powdered gold, treating breakage and repair as part of the history of an object, rather than something to disguise.'

I didn't want to hug the bruise of cancer any longer than I needed to, but I had to accept that living in the present was living with a healing body that was in transition. It was one that would always carry breakage and repair as part of its history, but Lowell's words hinted at the potential for that to be enriching rather than something to disguise.

It was interesting to have time on my hands. When I was a student, someone said to me that I would never again have as much free time in my life as I had then, while I was studying. Indignant, I refused to believe it, thinking myself so stressed and busy with my ten hours of lectures a week, and homework that I rarely did. But they were right. Life since had been a largely enjoyable, occasionally stressful, frequently hectic whirl of activity – of work, parenting, freelancing, more study, creativity, running, spirituality, friends, family and more.

Over the previous five months I'd had to slow down and finally I had come to an enforced stop. I had the luxury of paid time off work so I could concentrate on getting better, but it was strange to have no structure to my days unless I created one. I wasn't complaining, just observing that the free time and lack of responsibilities you crave when you are overwhelmed with the busyness of life looks different when it is all you have. I tried to settle into recovery being my main priority and to let go of the feeling that I ought to be achieving something.

This was the longest time I had spent without running for years. I missed it, of course, but I didn't trust my refigured body enough yet to try, and I was following the advice from my doctors who had said to wait at least six weeks. I got some of my running fix vicariously through watching what my clubmates were up to.

Then Julie e-mailed me from her holiday in Sweden where she went running and had a strong sense that I was running with her. She said, 'We ran together today through a forest of tall pine trees and it was wonderful. As we ran we saw so many beautiful things: an ant hill hiding between the trees; the lake glistening and shimmering in the sunlight; geese calling to each other as they took flight across the sky, a beautiful old tree lying across the forest floor. As we ran, I noticed the leaves changing colour from green to orange to brown, falling gently from the trees in the cycle of life. Autumn has to follow the abundance of summer; winter follows autumn when everything lies dormant, but spring will come and with it the promise of new life. May it be the same for you as you wait for your body to recover and new health to emerge.'

While my body was firmly in slow walking mode through London parks and streets, I loved the idea that I was somehow running with her in the wild, strong and free, along trails and under trees; it made sense to me at the time. Meanwhile, a silent, soft fuzz of hair was appearing, unbidden, on my head, a welcome sign that my body was doing what it should and things were going in the right direction.

Jonny and I went to see the oncologist to hear the results of the surgery. The cancer was grade one, which is the slowest-growing, and stage three because there was a relatively large tumour and it was in my lymph nodes. The chemotherapy had shrunk the main tumour to a third of its size, and they had found two smaller tumours in the breast, but they had been able to cut it all out with a clear margin of healthy cells. There was cancer in five of the lymph nodes they had removed, so although I could consider myself free of cancer after the surgery, the reality was that it had begun to spread from the original site and I would need to have regular monitoring and an annual mammogram for the foreseeable future. Overall it was relatively good news, and it certainly could have been a lot worse, but I was still holding on to the hope that this would all be over by Christmas, that cancer would be a thing in my past, and it was a blow to realise that hospital visits would continue to be a part of my life for years.

There was no going back to the sweet oblivion at the start of this year when cancer was something that happened to other people. The child within me whimpered 'they've made me ill and they can't make me better', which made no sense, but showed that deep down, I was still trying to come to terms with all of this. Radiotherapy would need to be delayed a bit because the skin on my new breast wasn't fully healed, which meant that it would run into Christmas. Back at home I e-mailed my boss to say that

I would not return to work this year after all, and he replied, 'Surgery is always much more than a physical thing and you need time to heal and to find yourself again.'

He was right. There are some things that you can watch heal. Wounds become scars that then slowly fade. Broken skin stops weeping and becomes smooth and pink again. But it was a mistake to think that everything was okay once the physical effects of surgery faded; there was a lot more unseen healing that needed to take place deep within, regaining confidence, learning to trust my body again.

I went for some counselling at The Haven in Fulham, a breast cancer support centre, and it was cathartic to talk to someone who didn't know me about what I had been through over the last few months. Jan Leach, a friend from my masters course, invited me to go to a Breast Cancer Now event with her. She had been raising money for research into breast cancer ever since her sister died of the disease several years before. She had nominated my name for a fundraising wall at the Institute of Cancer Research and we went to see it being unveiled.

I talked to one of the researchers there about the causes of cancer and found myself moved to tears when she said that cancer is a random event. I realised that deep down I thought I had brought this on myself in some way; so deep down that I had not appreciated that was a burden I was carrying until that conversation. Jan and I had lunch afterwards and I travelled home feeling grateful and loved. And then that evening I crashed into a deep despair, and went to bed feeling lost and broken.

Of course, I had had those kind of days at different points in my life before where I had gone from joy to gloom in the space of a few hours, perhaps most of us do, but the presence of illness somehow intensified it all because fear seeps in and you do not know whether you will ever find your way back to yourself again.

The next day I went down to Pickwell in Devon to take part in a social entrepreneurs' course, a structured week to help people who have an idea for bringing about social change to turn that into reality. I went partly because Pickwell is such a beautiful place and Susie and Steve were involved in running the week, and partly to think some more about a greeting card idea I had had a few months previously. Buying birthday cards for my nieces over the last few years had made me realise how stereotyped greetings cards could be.

Most cards aimed at girls were pink and focused on their appearance, or shopping or shoes, offering them a limited experience of life rather than encouraging them to fulfil their potential and explore the world. I wondered if there was another way of shaping that small intervention in a girl's life so that family and friends could encourage them to dream big, one that opened up opportunities rather than trying to squeeze them into a gender-stereotyped box. I arrived in Devon feeling withdrawn and slightly prickly, but actually it was just what I needed – an opportunity to focus on and talk about something creative and positive, to meet interesting and inspiring people, and for cancer to retreat to a whisper in the background rather than dominating the conversation.

As I recovered, I found the idea of 'practising' really helpful, as in the sense of actively working at a profession, or actively following a way of life. Practising is the doing of something whether you feel like it or not, in the expectation that what might seem strange at the beginning will eventually flow and become a natural part of who you are. So the practice of massaging oil into the scars on my abdomen and breast made me look at and touch my changed body, and although it didn't feel quite like 'me' yet, I trusted that the practice would get me there.

The practice of working on ideas with other entrepreneurs, when my confidence was wavering and I had forgotten what I was good at, put me in a place where I was expected to be creative and relate to other people, so of course I did and I could, which was a very healing thing. And like the dreadful clarinet practice I did as a child, it doesn't matter if you get it wrong as long as you keep doing it. It is not about being fake or about pushing yourself unhelpfully; it is having faith that this version of yourself is not permanent and acting accordingly.

I had arrived at the six-week post-surgery milestone so I went out for a run. In Devon I had enjoyed a five-mile walk through windswept sand dunes and along the beach, and so trying to run did not seem unreasonable. I did my two laps of the common, the benchmark that had shown me after each chemo treatment that I was getting my strength back. It was snowing as I ran, gentle flakes brushing my eyelids and disappearing as they hit the ground. It was such a delight to be back in my trainers, to be drinking in deep breaths of cold air even if it was tainted by the traffic clogging up the North Circular.

The run felt easy at the time, but the next day my right knee was quite sore. I did some strengthening exercises and spent time with my foam roller, and decided that I needed to be patient for just a bit longer. Clearly the surgery had had a bigger impact on my body and I had lost more fitness than I had realised. I reluctantly put my trainers back in the cupboard, but also decided that I needed to be more intentional about getting physically stronger. I went to see Rachel, my chiropractor, who said my pelvis had been pulled out of alignment again by the surgery and by not being able to stand up properly for over a fortnight; she straightened me out over the next few weeks. I signed up for a few one-to-one sessions with a personal trainer who slowly got my core muscles working again.

And I decided that I would give up my 2016 London Marathon place. I had registered for it back in July and had hoped that it could be my big comeback race after cancer treatment, proof that I was back to normal and everything was okay again. But a standard 16-week training plan would need to start at the beginning of January, just over a month away. If I couldn't even do two miles now, it would be a big stretch to get race-ready and it felt like an unnecessary pressure. If I was going to run a marathon again, I wanted to be able to run it well and I had to concede that the London Marathon in 2016 would be too much too soon.

However, I did start wondering whether there were other more reasonable targets I could aim for. At the end of November, I went to watch Lucy doing her 50th parkrun. Wrapped up warm against the cold wind, it was exhilarating to watch so many different people running and not for the first time I thought, 'This is my tribe.' There were so many familiar faces there, and it was great to catch up with people in the café afterwards. My friend Katie was doing her second parkrun after giving birth to her daughter Imogen in September, and Arlene, one of the founders of Gunnersbury parkrun, was doing it as part of her hen weekend in a white dress and veil surrounded by a posse of her friends.

When I had been thinking about how to celebrate my 50th birthday the previous March I had been aiming to do my 50th parkrun while I was still 50. I had got up to parkrun number 38 the week before the surgery and I started to do some maths. I worked out that if I did one the week before Christmas and if I took advantage of the extra parkruns that happen on Christmas Day and New Year's Day, then '50 while I'm 50' was still possible.

I also decided that I would try and qualify for the Eagles' club championships. I had won my age category the previous year and there was no way I would be able to do that again, not least because Jen Watt had moved up into the same age group as me and even at my fastest I was no match for her. But it would be pleasing to qualify and feature in the rankings even if I was last. The championship year would finish the following April and overall there were 20 races of different lengths, from a mile to a marathon. To qualify, you had to do seven out of the eight different types of race and your best five placings would be counted.

I had done three so far thanks to the Summer League races I had done during chemo and a parkrun in October just before surgery. I would need to do a half-marathon and a cross-country race in February, and then a ten-miler and a mile race in April. This too was possible. It was so important to me to be able to set myself these goals. I had always loved planning ahead, thinking about the next challenge, wanting to discover what I was capable of, delighting in some healthy competition. Since May the previous year that had largely been denied me, and I had had to let go of my plans one by one, each one reluctantly and with a sense of loss. I knew better than to bank on these new goals – I was going to hold them very lightly – but in making them it felt like I was reclaiming an important part of myself.

Three weeks after my first attempt, I tried another two laps of the common. This time, having been straightened out by Rachel and strengthened by the personal training sessions, I ran without any problems, a quiet achievement that brought me great joy.

I did a slightly longer run a couple of days later, so that I was ready the weekend before Christmas to do my 39th parkrun. I was one runner among hundreds, most of them dressed as Father Christmas because they were going on to do the Eagles' Santa Run straight afterwards. There must have been lots of people there for whom that parkrun was significant – perhaps their first, or their fastest, or the longest they had done without walking. I had never been so delighted to run 5k before. I went home for a hot shower, hugging this small victory to myself.

Each December for the last few years, I had put a summary of my running year on my blog in order to record and celebrate what I had done. The previous years had been all about the PBs I had run and my highest mileage ever. This year's was not about how far or how fast I had gone, but about the lifeline that running had been for me during a difficult 12 months.

I was hugely appreciative of the medical team who had taken me through the different stages of treatment with patience and understanding, particularly with the complications of my liver and the thrombophlebitis.

I was slightly in awe of my family and friends who had offered me such generous emotional and practical support, and made me realise that people loved me more than I ever knew.

But I was also so grateful for my running. In all that I had been through over the last nine months, running had been my companion, a source of life and hope and something that anchored me to who I truly was when I felt that I was losing my very self.

Who knew that putting on your trainers and getting out of the door could be so significant?

My Running Year 2015

This has now become a tradition, to look back at the end of the year in a spirit of celebration at all the running I have done. I didn't do the running I had planned to in 2015, but what I have done has been a lifeline.

I ran 853 miles, 580 of them before I started treatment in May.

I ran in just four races – Watford Half-Marathon, Palestine 10k and two summer league races in Perivale and Harrow. I did 20 parkruns, most of them at Gunnersbury but also at Bushy Park, Kingston, Wormwood Scrubs, Bath Skyline, Preston Park and Brighton. I marshalled at three races – Ealing Half-Marathon, Ealing 10k and Osterley 10k and volunteered at parkrun. Almost all of my running has been in and around Ealing, but I managed runs in North Devon, Herefordshire and Bath while we were on holiday in the summer, and some in Brighton this Christmas. I have had writing about running published on the *Guardian* running blog and in *Like the Wind* magazine. And I won the club championship prize for my age group in the 2014/15 season, just before I started chemotherapy.

Some runs that stand out:

- On my last long run before the Palestine Marathon in March, I fell in Richmond Park about nine miles into the run. I landed flat on my face and banged my knee really hard, but I needed to do 16 miles that day so I decided to run home. At Kew Bridge I was in so much pain that I rang Jonny to ask him to pick me up, at which point my phone ran out of battery, so I had to hobble the final two miles. I ended up having to withdraw from both the Palestine Marathon and London which felt catastrophic at the time, but in the wider context of this year seems really insignificant now.

- I still went to Palestine and ran the 10k instead, a chaotic, joyful, defiant celebration of life that still makes me smile when I think about it.

- My last run to work before I started treatment felt really poignant as I headed into the unknown of chemotherapy. I took photos as I ran, wanting to savour every moment and ran past the Household Cavalry parading in Hyde Park.

- I joined Tracey Melville for her 100th parkrun in September which I found really emotional, as she had treatment for cancer last year. I burst into tears as I crossed the line, and caused havoc with the tokens.

- My runs to chemo were so life-giving, from the second sorrowful one with Lucy to the final one that was such a celebration. Running to chemo meant that instead of dreading the treatment, I looked forward to the run. It meant that I arrived at the hospital in my trainers and on my terms. I am so grateful to all the people who ran with me.

In 2014 it was a year of PBs and I had a sense that it would be the year that I peaked. This year has not been about running faster or running further, but about running being a source of life, healing and normality, both in the actual running I have done but also in the amazing community of running friends who have sustained and encouraged me over the last few months.

Rather than setting myself too many running goals for next year, I will wait to see how it unfolds. I have deferred my London good-for-age place until 2017. I would love to do another marathon and try that ultra but I don't want to push myself to do too much too soon. Next year will be about running in beautiful places and savouring every moment.

How To Help

The end of the year is always a time for reflection, for looking back at what happened, remembering the best bits, observing how you got through the worst, but especially so this year. Ten weeks on from my surgery I feel like I am coming back to myself, and I can draw breath, lift my head up from the tension of recovery and take stock.

Cancer doesn't just happen to the person who discovers it is in their body; it happens to their family and friends, more intensely the closer to the person they are. I think it is hard for those around us to know how to help or what to do particularly when they are coping with their own pain at what is happening, and so I wanted to write about how people have supported me, to honour what they have done and in case it is helpful to anyone else.

There is no hierarchy in the list that follows; sometimes the smallest things had an enormous impact. There is no guarantee that something you do for someone with cancer will have the effect you hoped; there were times when I felt so rubbish that I couldn't summon the energy to look enthusiastic or even text a thank you.

But I had to trust that what was offered was done in a true spirit of generosity, not done to meet the needs of the giver. A true gift does not ask for anything in return. Someone wisely said to me, 'People aren't helping you, unless *you* think they're helping.' There were times, particularly after surgery, when people wanted to visit and I turned them down because I needed to hide away and get better. My people-pleasing tendencies have had to be overshadowed by self-preservation which is no bad thing.

I found writing on my blog a very positive thing. It helped me process what was going on and it also meant people knew the basics of what was happening; I didn't have to keep updating people with how my treatment was going. I found

I didn't mind talking about it when people asked me how I was, although it was also a relief to get caught up in other things and for cancer to recede into the background. But not everyone chooses to go public with their diagnosis; not everyone can because of the impact it might have on their work; not everyone wants to talk about it.

As I have said before there is no blueprint for how to cope with cancer. What I found helpful might not suit your friend who has just had a diagnosis; we need to work these things out for ourselves, but hopefully because you know her, you will also know how to show her that you are with her in what she is facing. And sometimes there is nothing anyone can do to help, but it is still important to be there. Because of regular periods of chemo brain and the intensity of surgery, I may have forgotten some of the things people did for me, so if your contribution is not on this list, please don't take it personally. So after all those caveats, this is what helped me:

- People have sent me a constant supply of cards and flowers from the time I was diagnosed, to after my operation. I was really touched to know that people hadn't forgotten what I was going through, even though it was going on for months. A few people sent me cards regularly, so even though I have not seen them in person I know they have been with me through all that has happened.

- Contact with people through social media has been brilliant. So many people have read my blog, and interacted there or on Facebook or Twitter. Every 'like', retweet, or comment, every text or e-mail has given me a very real sense that people are in this with me. When I was first diagnosed, I felt I had been transported into a strange land where I didn't know my way around and I didn't know the rules. People getting in touch felt like they were choosing to enter this new space with me.

- Friends remembered my change of diet which meant a lot. Lots of people sent me dark chocolate or vegan snacks. A couple of people bought me recipe books, and one friend sent me some family recipes. One friend cooked me a vegan supper and brought it round. I didn't feel like socialising much, but some lovely friends invited us round regularly and didn't mind if I fell asleep on the sofa or had nothing much to say.

- A friend went through treatment for infertility a few years ago. She was given a tin of gifts entitled a 'Human Repair Kit'. She gave the tin to me full of gorgeous things like homemade hand scrub, dark chocolate and lavender from her garden along with a card from her daughter. I loved the idea that the love she had been shown in her darkest time was now being passed on to me. I will look out for someone that I can hand it on to in the future.

- Friends bought me gifts for my less active days, knowing that I would need help to fill them – books to read, knitting, colouring, sudoku puzzles.

- A friend had her hair cut in sympathy with my baldness, donating it to the Little Princess Trust to be made into a wig for children with cancer, and raising money in the process.

- A friend in my running club is known as Bald Eagle. The Order of the Bald Eagle is an award given to club members who have run a marathon in under three hours if they are men or under 200 minutes for women. He sent me a framed certificate admitting me as an extraordinary member of the Order in recognition of my 'fashionable baldness and regular training runs to Charing Cross Hospital'. I was so touched. There is no way on earth I would qualify for this OBE in normal circumstances; it was very pleasing to sneak into this exclusive club through the back door.

HOW TO HELP

- A friend bought me a long-sleeved t-shirt after my operation, so that I would have something soft to wear against my skin. I could only wear a very few of my clothes straight after the op and had no energy to go shopping, so this meant a lot.

- My sister sent me a headband just as I was starting chemo which I wore most of the time during the summer. And a couple of weeks ago a friend sent me a woolly hat to wear which is just right for this weather; even though I do have some hair now, it is not enough to keep my head warm.

- My nose ran a lot when I lost my hair and I never remembered to take tissues with me, so was constantly sniffing. One friend had tissues for me every time I saw her and offered them without comment. Little things like a clean tissue on a cold day make such a difference.

- A friend gave me 'kudos' on Strava every time I went out for a run, even if it was just a couple of miles. It was a small acknowledgement that touched me at home, and made me feel seen.

So thank you to everyone who has been there for me in all these different ways over the last few months, and all those I have forgotten. You have made all the difference and I don't know what I would have done without you.

9

Radiotherapy

Mid-December to Early January

ADVENT is a time of year that has always had lots of resonance for me and it seemed particularly poignant this year as I slowly regained my strength and my sense of self after surgery. Advent is the season of waiting, and of longing for restoration. It is a time infused with darkness when we get up before the sun and go to bed long after it has disappeared, the shortest day being the turning point for the journey back to the light. It was a warm December and confused trees were producing unseasonal blossom, a reminder that it doesn't take much for new life to appear.

The stream of cards, messages and e-mails that had been triggered by my diagnosis had slowed down but still hadn't stopped. I spent a weekend re-reading these expressions of love and support and sticking them into an album, wanting to honour and hold on to them for the days when I knew I would forget them. Through the disbelief of the diagnosis, the fog of chemo, the shock of surgery and the slow days of recovery that followed, they had been a means of people drawing alongside me and keeping me company even if they were not physically present.

RADIOTHERAPY

It is hard to know what to do when someone you love is having a tough time, but what matters is that you do something. Getting a card, an e-mail or a text had had a bigger impact on me than the person who sent it probably expected. I wrote at the beginning of the album, 'People love you more than you know', and hoped that that truth would penetrate through my insecurities and take root somewhere deep within.

It was a relief to be approaching the end of all the treatment, but after the drama of chemotherapy and the shock of surgery, radiotherapy was a strangely impersonal and soulless experience. I went for an initial scan at the end of November where they mapped out exactly where they would target the rays. I was given three tiny tattoo spots so they could line me up in exactly the same position under the machine each time, one in the centre of my chest and one under each armpit. I would need 15 daily sessions of radiotherapy starting in the middle of December and carrying on over Christmas, finishing in the New Year.

Having experienced over an hour's wait for the scan, I asked for early morning appointments for the treatment to try and get seen before the inevitable delays built up; I didn't want to have to spend any more time in hospital than I had to.

Harry came with me to my first session. We cycled there, setting off in the stillness before sunrise and following the north bank of the river, the opposite side to where we had run in the summer, because the route was mainly roads and smoother than the bumpy path on the south side. I have always loved cycling in the dark through quiet streets at either end of the day, using my own strength to get myself from one place to another. This was a slow cycle, savouring the cold morning air, enjoying the feeling of being outdoors, drawing it out to make it last and pushing the reason for the ride to the back of my mind for as long as possible.

We locked up our bikes outside the hospital and reported to reception. I changed into the hospital gown I had been given to use throughout the treatment and sat waiting to be called. I completely understood why I should just use one gown over the next three weeks. It was a waste of resources to do anything else when I would wear it for less than ten minutes each day, but I hated its pattern, its shapelessness, its ribbons that were so fiddly to tie together and all that it stood for. Carting it around in my bag every day was an unwelcome reminder that I was a patient.

When it was my turn, I followed a nurse into the radiotherapy room and lay on the bench, naked from the waist up, with my arms in supports above my head. The radiographers needed to make sure I was in exactly the right position on the bench, so they pushed my body this way and that, and read out measurements to each other over me while I tried to stay as still as possible. They left the room while the radiotherapy happened, leaving me feeling vulnerable and isolated, and very cold. The heavy machine rotated around me, buzzing and whirring and clicking, moving closer and pulling away. Then a few minutes later it was done; time for me to leave and for them to move on to the next patient.

I don't know that it could be done any differently; I wanted the radiographers to focus on getting my treatment right, not chat to me about whether I had seen any good films lately. They were there to do their job and to do it well, not to be my mate. But it was a detached and lonely experience, particularly as I rarely saw the same member of staff from one day to the next.

It helped that there was Christmas to celebrate in the middle of it all, and a few days' respite because of bank holidays and the weekend. Jonny and I went down to Brighton to stay with his mum and see his family. While we were there we did Preston Park parkrun on Christmas Day, which sparked fond memories of the Brighton Marathon I had done a few years before which starts in the same place. And then on Boxing Day we did Brighton and Hove parkrun in Hove Park.

Jonny would never call himself a runner, and he had had to put up with people from my club trying to convert him at every social event we had been to over the last few years. He was more of a team sportsman and used to play a lot of basketball, cricket and football when he was younger but opportunities to do that seem to disappear as you get older. I was touched that he wanted to do parkrun with me, perhaps to keep an eye on me and to make sure that I made it round in one piece.

Back in London I kept cycling to my appointments, counting down the days to the end. Each visit followed the same tedious pattern: wait to be called; change into that unattractive hospital gown; follow a nurse into a room full of mysterious machinery; bare your upper body while trying to hold on to your dignity; lie down on the narrow bench with your arms above your head; surrender yourself to being manoeuvred into place; listen to numbers being called out over you; trust the radiographers to get the settings just right; lie there alone as the machine moves around you, choosing to believe that this strange experience is making a difference; get the go-ahead to leave; tick off one more treatment on the list in your head.

I didn't run much during radiotherapy because the treatment can make your skin sore and inflamed, like sunburn, and I knew that covering the area with a sports bra and then getting hot and sweaty would not help. I did clock up a couple more parkruns, though. I cycled to Richmond Park on New Year's Day and slowly made my way round the course. I was beaten by a woman running with twins in a double buggy but I was delighted just to be there and to add one more run to my total. That afternoon we drove to Ely to stay with my mum, ready for belated Christmas celebrations with my side of the family the next day. We headed up early so that I could do Cambridge parkrun on the Saturday morning with my sister Susie. Arriving at my mum's, I discovered that I had left my running shoes behind. Normally they were the first thing I packed every time I went away and I could not believe I had forgotten them. I blamed it on 'chemo brain' and fortunately was able to borrow a pair of trainers from my nephew Jake.

Cambridge parkrun is in Milton Country Park, created on the site of old gravel pits, and is run on trails around the lakes. There were nearly 400 runners that morning, and the narrow paths meant that once you had found your pace, you mostly stayed in sequence because it was too tricky to try and pass people. It was a grey drizzly morning but it was fun to slosh through mud, dodge tree roots, and breathe in the earthy smell of the countryside. Jake came in first out of the three of us, of course. We headed back to my mum's for showers and hot coffee, before spending the day eating and drinking, her house full of family.

Ever since Joel and Harry were little, we had spent an evening each New Year doing a bittersweet reflection together. We would look back over the year that had just gone, and talk about the things that had happened that had been bitter or sad, writing them on a big sheet of paper on the table between us. We would then do the same for our sweet memories of the previous year.

Sometimes, particularly when they were younger, we ate lemon slices, and honey with breadsticks to accompany the different shades of the ritual, matching abstract emotions with familiar flavours; always we would give thanks for God's presence through all that had happened. This year we did the same, joined by Kat and Grace, Harry's girlfriend. Once again I was reminded how privileged we were because even in this year where cancer dominated the bitter conversation, there were so many sweet things to more than balance it out – graduations, travel, friends, seeing Joel, Kat, Harry and Grace immersed in interesting work that enabled them to do what they loved, and not least, the birth of beautiful Florence.

We wrote our hopes and dreams for the year ahead on paper and made them into origami birds, perhaps to encourage us to give wings to those stirrings within. I found myself hesitant to write down any big plans or ideas for the year beyond having a haircut, growing my nails long enough to have a manicure and finding a bra that fitted. My plans for 2015 were cut off in their prime, but it had still been a year of rich experiences and powerful relationships. My instinct was to get stronger, get back to work and see what happened from there.

The final week of radiotherapy arrived. I had discovered some spots on my back when I had got home after the treatment on Friday the week before so I asked one of the nurses to have a look at them. I thought perhaps I had developed a rash because the bench had not been cleaned properly, but it turned out I had shingles, an annoying complication to have to cope with on top of everything else, and a sign of the battering my immune system was under. I was given some anti-viral medication and told to take things easy.

I took the tube to my appointment the next day, but then cycled again with Harry on the Wednesday, convinced that these slow cycles were more life-giving than anything else, that they were energising rather than depleting. Being at hospital every weekday for three weeks had put me firmly in the role of being a patient, where my primary identity was as someone who needed to be fixed. It was easy to be passive and to feel diminished, whereas the simple act of cycling to hospital made me feel more myself and more in control.

And then it was the last one. I had arrived at the end of my treatment for cancer, weary but relieved that it was over. I endured the routine for one last time and then ditched my hospital gown in the laundry bin with delight and cycled home from the hospital along the river with a strong sense of leaving something behind and moving on. Of course, I already had more hospital appointments lined up and hormone therapy still to go, but the end of active treatment felt like a significant milestone, a line in the sand.

I no longer had the expectation that my experience of cancer would one day be 'over'. It had helped me to compare the treatment to running a race, but I had to face the fact that there was no finishing line and there would be no medal. There was no doctor telling me I was all right now and waving me a cheery goodbye. But I did feel a sense of achievement. I was coming out the other side of treatment a stronger person and a more grateful one. This past year had shown me that I could meet difficulty with creativity, determination, resilience, and a strong cast of family and friends around me.

I don't think I am particularly remarkable in that. So many people have to deal with cancer themselves, or in those they love, and lots of people have so much more to deal with than I had. When faced with a challenge like this, we dig deep to find the strength we need to get through the next thing. Sometimes we are surprised by the courage and determination we find. Other times we discover there is nothing left to draw on, but that people are there to catch us if we will let them.

My experience had made me look at myself in a different light and I wanted to try and hold on to that. I read an article in *The Guardian* about Victoria Pendleton, the Olympic cyclist, who that year had taken up horse racing. She talked about the training she was doing and how her trainer, Yogi, had told her that she had a lot of courage. She says, 'Yogi has used the word "courageous" a lot and I've never considered myself as having courage. But now that he's given it to me I want to keep it because courage is a word that defines this challenge.'

I liked that idea of keeping words that had been used about you. I wanted to keep all the positive things that people had said about me that year, to own those words more, because my default position was so often to feel the opposite. She went on to say, 'It really got me thinking that we all have access to courage. It's within us all and you can choose whether to be courageous or not. We've all said, "No, no I couldn't do that." But actually you could if you just went, "You know what? I will and I shall."'

What I needed courage for now was to re-enter my old life. Bizarrely, I had got quite comfortable being a cancer patient. I knew how to do it, to have my days driven by hospital appointments and a treatment plan. I liked being the centre of attention and to be thought of as heroic just for getting through the day. Of course, thinking rationally, I didn't want to stay in the world of cancer for any longer than I needed to, but I had to admit it had become my normal. Now radiotherapy was over, my New Year's task was to find my way back into my old life as I went back to work.

But first it was time to celebrate. It seemed important to mark the end of treatment and so I threw a party at the local pub and invited everyone who had been involved in some way or another over the previous nine months. Cancer has its own gravitational pull and it has an impact on everyone who comes into its orbit.

Cancer had happened to me, obviously, but it had also happened to everyone around me to a greater or lesser extent and I wanted to acknowledge that by inviting people to enjoy this ending with me.

The Prosecco flowed and there was live music from Chris Read and his band. Chris was a close friend of Harry's and I had known the band members since they were at primary school. Their infectious energy and musical skill got people dancing, and Harry joined them for a rendition of Black Eyed Peas' 'Let's Get It Started', going to town on the 'runnin', runnin', runnin'' refrain.

There were people there from so many different parts of my life: my running club of course, but also friends from work, church, and those I had got to know in the school playground when Joel and Harry were younger. Sheenagh and Richard Burrell had come to celebrate with me. Their son Simon was Joel's best friend and had been his best man at his wedding. Over the years, Joel and Simon had gone to school and to Boys' Brigade together, they had played football, formed a DJing partnership and recorded music as a duo called Twotone, and so the lives of our two families had overlapped and intertwined at different points.

Years before, Sheenagh and Richard's eldest son Edd had collapsed on a bus shortly after he started his music degree in York. After tests, they got the devastating news that he had a brain tumour and over the next few months they accompanied him through intensive treatment while we tried to be supportive from a distance, welcoming Simon into our family activities as much as was appropriate to provide a bit of respite. I remember calling round to see them around Christmastime that year; Sheenagh told us that they had just heard there was nothing more that could be done for Edd, and just a few weeks later, he died aged just 20.

It had been nine months since his diagnosis and at his funeral Sheenagh poignantly compared the nine months she had carried him in her womb with the time it had taken to accompany him to the end of his life, surely the hardest thing for any parent to have to do. I discovered at my party that it was the exact anniversary of his death, 11 years before. Although Sheenagh and Richard were still mourning the loss of their beautiful boy, they were there on the same day to mark the very different outcome of my entanglement with cancer.

When you get diagnosed with cancer you join a tribe of people that you would never choose to belong to, but where you find companionship and an understanding that does not need to be expressed in words. You don't ever get to leave but with my treatment over, I was aware that I was one of the more fortunate members.

Other people who I knew faced more complicated diagnoses, or had been told that their cancer was terminal. Many, many people, like the Burrells, had lost family and friends to the disease and would always carry the pain of their loss. I was mindful of my friends who were living with ME or other illnesses where treatment is not straightforward and there is no recovery in sight. Part of me had wondered whether it was insensitive to celebrate when others were not in that same place, but I knew that when any of my friends got to this kind of milestone I was delighted for them.

Sheenagh and Richard coming to my party was a powerful demonstration that this cancer tribe knows how to weep with those who weep, and rejoice with those who rejoice. And for me, now was a time for rejoicing.

10

Getting Myself Back

February to April

THE evening before my final radiotherapy session, I felt fed up and restless. I had spent a lot of time on my own that week, trying to follow the advice to rest and not do too much, and I was feeling out of sorts. I realised that what I was craving was the type of carefree running that I used to do before all this began.

So I went out in the rain, ignoring the need to be sensible, and just ran, picking up the pace from my usual careful jog until I was breathing hard and my feet were pounding the pavement. I ran beside the North Circular road and found myself shouting 'I want myself back' at the darkening sky, not really caring if there was anyone around to hear me. I followed the familiar route of my club run that I had done so many times before, running along streets, past shops and allotments, parks and churches. It was a hard run but it was cathartic and energising and I arrived home out of breath and smiling. I was tired of being tentative and careful, of feeling like I couldn't trust my body. I wanted myself back.

A few days later, I went bra shopping. Surgery had left me lopsided and I had been wearing a sports bra since October. At the beginning that was to keep my new breast supported and protected, but once it had recovered I actually didn't have any choice. My old bras just didn't fit and radiotherapy had made my skin quite tender so shopping for new ones had not been a priority until it was over. I had had conversations with Jude Hunter, my plastic surgeon, about 'symmetry surgery', which would reduce the size of my left breast and lift it so it matched the reconstructed one on the right. I could also have a reconstructed nipple or one tattooed on to the smooth surface of the reconstruction if I wanted.

After much thought I had decided not to have any of those. After my experience a few months before, I didn't want to have any more surgery than I absolutely needed. My left breast was healthy and I wanted to leave it as it was, not treat it as something that needed to be fixed just because my right breast had been altered. And even the most lifelike reconstructed nipple would not restore my new breast to what it had been before. It is a very personal choice and women will feel very differently about further surgery, but that felt right for me.

Now that the reconstruction had settled down and the scars were beginning to fade I was pleased with how it looked, and could at last feel grateful for what Jude and her team had done. I had never been one to flash my cleavage, but thanks to their skilful surgery at least I still had some cleavage to show if I ever felt the need to put it on display.

However, I was desperate to ditch the daily wearing of my sports bra. Essential as they are when you are running, sports bras are restrictive and hot when you wear them every day and their high, thick straps were visible above the neckline of a lot of my clothes, another daily reminder of what had happened.

I went to a specialist mastectomy bra shop in central London, the type of shop that you would never know existed unless you have been inducted into the world of breast cancer. A lovely shop assistant put me at ease and measured me, producing some bras that fitted me. She left me in the changing room while she packaged them up and I quietly dissolved in tears of relief, and then sobbed some more when I went to pay. Somehow having a bra that evened up my breasts, even if it was with a bit of padding, made me feel so much better and more myself.

I went back to work ten days after radiotherapy finished, on a phased return working part-time until Easter. My colleagues gave me a lovely welcome; there were cards and flowers on my desk and homemade vegan truffles. It was good to see everyone again and I soon got back into the familiar routine of fighting a never-ending tide of e-mails and visiting the partnerships I managed around the country.

The final stage in my treatment was to be hormone therapy. The cancer had been found to be double positive, which meant that it contained receptors that bind to the hormones oestrogen and progesterone. The oestrogen in particular stimulated the cancer to grow and so it was important to try and stop that happening. I needed to take Tamoxifen, a drug that would block the effect of oestrogen on the receptors and help to stop any lingering breast cancer cells from multiplying. I had not been keen on taking it, having heard many stories of unwelcome side-effects.

I wanted to know exactly what difference it was going to make to me, which is an impossible thing to assess. However, the NHS has an online tool called Predict where you can input the details of your particular breast cancer diagnosis and it will tell you the prognosis for women who had treatment for the same thing, based on the outcomes of thousands of women in the UK. It told me that for women with a similar diagnosis and treatment plan, an additional eight per cent of those who took Tamoxifen were alive ten years later compared to those who did not, which felt significant enough to give it a go. I started taking it at the beginning of February, the first tablet on the first day to make it easy to remember. It made me feel nauseous for the first couple of weeks but that soon settled down. However, it also significantly increased the hot flushes I had been having for the last few months.

Chemotherapy pushes you into menopause with all its accompanying symptoms. At 50, I was probably nearly there anyway but since chemo started I hadn't had a period and I had been having around ten hot flushes a day. They started as a flu-like feeling from deep within, and then I would gradually get incredibly hot, as if someone had turned on an electric bar heater right next to me. Sometimes they were mild but more often they would bring me out in a real sweat which trickled down my neck, arms and back. When they subsided I was left cold and damp, until the next one. I had always hated being cold and loved to wrap up warm but I found I now needed to wear far less than I would naturally choose to try and make the flushes more manageable, and consequently I was permanently chilly. I got used to taking layers on and off multiple times during the day, and opening and closing windows to try and regulate my temperature.

Tamoxifen doubled the frequency of the flushes and I also started waking up three or four times in the night with them. Fortunately I woke each time just as I started to get hot, rather than waking in damp, sweaty bedding after they had happened. I would throw off the duvet and lie there until they subsided a couple of minutes later, but having such disturbed nights left me tired and annoyed. Over the next few weeks I tried acupuncture from two different practitioners, which is one treatment that some women have found effective, but that made little difference. I gave up coffee and ginger, and tried drinking sage tea to no effect. Alcohol did make the flushes a bit more severe, but I had cut that down anyway and I didn't want to sacrifice my remaining occasional glass of red wine.

Friends reminded me that menopause was a natural stage in a woman's life and to be welcomed, but since mine had been induced so fiercely by one set of chemicals and was being amplified by another I found it difficult to be so gracious. I found the flushes embarrassing, frustrating, invasive and debilitating by turn but there was nothing more I could do except endure them.

Meanwhile I was slowly building up my mileage again with an eye on the Wokingham Half-Marathon towards the end of February, one of the club championship races that I was determined to do. The weekend after my end of radiotherapy therapeutic stomp, my longest run was a seven-mile loop along the river. The following week I did eight miles, the furthest distance I had run since the previous July when I had had to give up on my dream of running the Ealing Half, and then managed ten miles the weekend after that. These were slow, solid, steady miles that were not trying to be anything more than extending the distance I could run, but I felt like I was getting back on track with my running.

I went to stay the weekend with Letty, who had prompted me to do my first marathon all those years before. She and her husband Dave took me to do the Long Eaton parkrun on Saturday morning in the rain, my 48th and my fastest since surgery. I loved spending time with Letty but I couldn't help comparing my previous year to hers; she had turned 50 like me, had had a creative and enriching sabbatical in Canada and now had an interesting new job which would stretch her in good ways. In contrast, I had been diagnosed with cancer and had had to let go of all the things I had hoped to achieve. There was no point in asking why; it was an impossible question. She wasn't being rewarded; I wasn't being punished. She had had her own different experiences of difficulty and sadness over the years, like so many people, and this was not Life Top Trumps with cancer holding the most points for the 'suffering' category.

The temptation to feel sorry for myself was still there. I tried to resist it because I knew it wouldn't get me anywhere, and it wasn't fair to her. I wanted to be pleased for her, not envious, to stay connected not pull away. I was trying to pay attention to these kind of feelings, naming and questioning them before they took root and festered. Getting back to health was not just about getting my physical strength back or being able to run long distances again, but looking after my heart and soul as well. I did not want the legacy of this year to be bitterness and resentment. I realised more than ever before that I needed my friends, and I didn't want to let toxic feelings come between us and keep us apart.

On Valentine's Day I joined the Eagles at a cross-country race in Royston, part of the Sunday League held at five different locations north of London each year. I had done this race a couple of years ago during my first season of cross-country. I had been apprehensive beforehand about trying this different type of running, my only other experience having been at school many years before where we ran across ridged fields in embarrassing athletic shorts and flimsy plimsolls, but I had quickly fallen in love with it.

According to Mark Rowlands in *Running with the Pack*, running is the very definition of play because its only true end is itself, and cross-country running was the epitome of playful running in my opinion, particularly when it was muddy and wet. I had fond memories of the South of England Cross Country Championships at Parliament Hill two years before where it had rained on already soggy ground, and the multitudes of runners churned up large parts of the course into a liquid mudbath. In places we were running ankle deep in chocolatey sludge and there was no choice but to surrender to getting completely soaked and covered in mud; that run for me was all about the experience rather than the competition because the conditions were so different to my usual running.

Royston wasn't muddy this year but my relative lack of fitness took any remaining sense of competition away. I was there just to participate and enjoy it. I walked up most of the hills and trotted down the other side, pleased to be out with my clubmates and to be earning more points for the championship. There were only 14 female Eagles taking part that day, so this became my highest-scoring race of the year, not because I was fast but because not many people turned up.

The following Saturday was my 50th parkrun. I had enjoyed squeezing parkruns in where I could over the previous couple of months and I had added six new locations to my parkrun tourism. Azariah came to run it with me, along with Jonny, Lucy and several other friends. Some of my friends who couldn't make it to Ealing did their local parkrun instead, Susie and her family in Cambridge, Letty and Dave in Long Eaton among others. Harry and Grace were travelling in Australia at the time and they went out for a run through a park in Melbourne to celebrate with me, texting me a photo as proof.

There were a couple of other people at Gunnersbury doing their 50th or 100th run that week so it was not hugely remarkable in the grand scheme of things, but it had helped me to have something to aim for and it was fun to celebrate another milestone just six weeks after finishing radiotherapy. I had made cupcakes with lurid red icing and '50' piped on top which I handed out to runners, marshals and spectators, anyone who had contributed to the morning in some way.

Hot on the heels of my '50 while I'm 50' parkrun came the Wokingham Half-Marathon the following day. I drove Lucy and a couple of friends over and we met a posse of Eagles near the start line in Cantley Park. I was being evasive about what time I was aiming for, telling people that I just wanted to finish, but secretly I wanted to come in under two hours. The race wound out of the park and across a bridge over the M4 before snaking through country lanes and villages, and doubling back on itself to finish where it started.

A few Eagles had come to cheer on the runners and take photos, their smiling faces a welcome encouragement out on the route. It was a flat course and I managed a fairly consistent nine-minute mile pace for most of it, but towards the end I really felt my lack of consistent training. Approaching the finish line, the last stretch of the race found us running into a headwind, and I dropped to a walk, feeling exhausted. Another runner touched me on the arm and said, 'Keep going, you're nearly there!', turning to smile at me and give me a cheer when I started running again. That was all I needed, the kindness of a stranger, and I crossed the line in 1 hour 57 minutes.

It was the same time that I had done in my first half-marathon in Folkestone six years before. Cancer had effectively wiped out six years of training and progress. It was a bit of a reality check to see just how much fitness I had lost. While I had been having treatment, new people had joined the club and almost everyone else seemed to have got faster. There were lots of PBs that day, including one for Lucy who finished a few seconds outside 1 hour 45. I was really pleased for her but it made me realise that I would have a lot of work to do if I were ever to improve on my times of a couple of year previously. For now, it was enough to have run the distance and have finished well. Getting faster again could wait.

Back at home, after a long, hot shower and a welcome lunch, I went public with my sponsorship page for the Palestine Half-Marathon in April. Now that I had run Wokingham Half, I knew that I would be able to do it again in slightly more challenging conditions in another six weeks or so. I had signed up and booked my flights the night before my surgery back in October, a deliberate act of faith that I would be able to run it the following year, while also acknowledging that I didn't expect to be back to full marathon form by then. It would be the fourth year I had taken part and, having done the marathon and the 10k, it was quite pleasing to be completing the hat-trick of distances on offer.

Over the previous few months I had got to know two other women who had had treatment for breast cancer at a similar time to me and who had also signed up for the race, Su McClellan and Helen Powell. Su worked for Embrace, a charity supporting transformation in the Middle East, and Helen was a long-term supporter of theirs. We had connected via Facebook and were all going to raise money for Al-Ahli Hospital in Gaza. The differences in treatment and prognosis for Gazan women and for us had stayed with me ever since learning about them from Chris's trip the previous May, and had challenged me whenever I felt my treatment was too much to endure; I was having the treatment I needed as soon as I needed it so who was I to complain?

Gaza is smaller than the Isle of Wight and is home to 1.8 million people, making it one of the most densely populated places on the planet. Al-Ahli Hospital has been running a breast cancer programme for the last five years and screens 1,200 women a year, but while they offer the very best care they can, they are hampered by heightened demand, scarce resources and limited equipment. They have good surgical facilities for breast surgery, but for women who need either chemotherapy or hormone therapy, there is no guarantee of finishing it as stocks of the drugs often run out.

And there are no facilities at all in Gaza for radiotherapy so women have to apply for permission to travel, to Jerusalem, Jordan or Egypt. One doctor had told Su, 'Very often by the time the necessary permissions arrive for patients to travel it is not about cure, it is about palliative care.' I had been able to cycle to most of my radiotherapy sessions, choosing what transport I took depending on how I felt on the day. Women in Gaza deserved better.

Asking for sponsorship is my least favourite aspect of running. Over the years I had done it lots of times for different causes and it had enabled me to raise thousands of pounds but I had always felt slightly uncomfortable about it. This year, that discomfort seemed a small price to pay, and Su, Helen and I had a great story – women who had had breast cancer raising money for women with breast cancer. I think all of us wanted to wring every last good thing we could out of our experience, and make it count for something bigger than just us. The donations started trickling in, along with lovely messages of support and encouragement from people who had already been so generous to me with their time and their love.

I was enjoying getting back into running, but deep down I was struggling. I was going through the motions at work but I didn't feel on top of things, and I was lacking in motivation. I felt frustrated with myself that I was not back to normal, able to do all that I had been doing a year ago but, with hindsight, my expectations of myself were far too high and I had gone back to work far too soon after the end of my treatment. That was nobody's fault but my own; there was no pressure from my boss and although I had used up all my sick pay, we could have managed for longer without me earning money.

I had not had any advice about going back to work from the various medical people I had seen, but I could have asked more questions and found out what other people did. Bizarrely, I found myself nostalgic for the predictability of chemotherapy and I indulged myself with wistful and very selective memories of the previous summer when I had had lots of time to write and think and mooch about. I think what I was doing was similar to the experience of running a marathon, or giving birth. Straight after the first time you swear you will never do it again, but a few weeks or months later the memory of the pain has faded and you are planning the next one. Of course I didn't want to have to go through chemotherapy again, I really didn't, but there was something about the structure and passivity of that time that appealed to me. I didn't have to make decisions; I didn't have to accomplish anything; I just had to turn up in the right place at the right time and have things done to me.

The sense of achievement I felt after radiotherapy had finished had been real and I still experienced those feelings from time to time, but at other moments I felt incredibly bleak. Cancer treatment had brought an intensity and a focus to life, stripping away all that was peripheral or superficial, and I felt I had lost something when it had ended. I couldn't help feeling that I should have had some kind of an epiphany and that my life should be dramatically better because I had survived the trial of cancer; instead it was the same old life that I was now struggling with.

I felt that cancer had spat me out in the same place I had been a year ago, but with a shakier core and less confidence to cope with it. I'd had a privileged life which I had taken completely for granted, and I had always assumed that it would continue in the same vein but now that assumption seemed incredibly naïve; how could I expect anything good to happen in the future?

I was still hanging on to my faith in God by my flaky fingernails but I found it impossible to pray for myself. Every so often I would get stuck in this cycle of thoughts, and find myself spiralling down into a sense of deep despair which left me feeling lost and broken. I found it really hard to admit my weakness and to ask for help; somehow I felt that I should be coping better. But I did talk to Jonny and to a couple of close friends. Articulating my darkest thoughts somehow took the power out of them and gave me a bit of perspective.

The counsellor I had seen a few weeks before had warned me to expect continuing aftershocks from the epicentre of the cancer diagnosis; even all these months later I was still grieving and coming to terms with it all. Julie Johnson talked to me about self-compassion which I found helpful and I realised that I needed to be more intentional about looking after my mental health. I could choose to practise gratitude, to be kind to myself, and to give myself a break. I needed to recalibrate my expectations. Recovering from something like cancer is not a nice straight line from 'ill' to 'better', but an undulating, complicated, messy process that touches body, mind and spirit, that goes backwards and forwards unpredictably and that takes a lot longer than you expect.

Our holiday the previous summer had been dominated by chemotherapy and hospitals and so Jonny and I treated ourselves to a week in Iceland over half-term. We rented a small apartment in Reykjavik and hired a car so that we could explore. It was the end of winter so there was still snow on the ground, but not too much to make travelling around difficult. The startling landscapes and wide-open skies did my soul good and I found it a place where I could breathe deeply and start to relax again.

I went running of course. I love travelling, but arriving in a foreign city always leaves me slightly on edge. Strange streets, an unfamiliar language on street signs, a different style of architecture all serve to remind me that I do not belong here. Almost imperceptibly, my mind stays on alert to stop me getting lost or breaking the local rules. Gradually over the next few days I know that I will find my way and begin to sink into my surroundings, learning to read the space and the people around me. And running always helps to kick-start that process.

On our first morning in Reykjavik, I went for a run through dark streets and out towards the sea. I had pored over a map of the city the night before and I had a vague understanding of its layout in my head as I ran. Running turns lines on a map into places you know; the act of marking the streets with your feet draws them into your experience and builds your mental picture of where you are.

The moments you invest in exploring the city reward you with a sense of familiarity and permission to relax. There is something about being and breathing in a space that begins to make it your own. But unlike a touristy stroll, running asks for nothing in return. When I am running, I am running. I don't need to be entertained or see sights or consume culture. I am just doing what I love, offering myself to this new place, setting out with a general sense of where I want to go, trusting the map in my head to get me back to where I started and knowing that I have a phone in my pocket if I do get lost.

I ran along the waterfront towards the light along the horizon which indicated where the sun would soon appear. There was snow on the ground that had been there for a while; the centre of the path had been compacted by feet to an icy hardness. My trail shoes crunched in a satisfying way as I ran, head bent into the wind, fists clenched against the cold. I arrived back at the flat with a sense of accomplishment at having found my way around and with a different kind of knowledge of this new place.

We explored Reykjavik on foot and in the afternoon went to a swimming pool in Laugardalur in the centre of the city. We wanted to experience the natural hot water that Iceland is famous for and this seemed like a good place to start. We paid to get in and split up to get changed, agreeing to meet in the pool in five minutes' time.

Walking into the female changing rooms I was confronted by a poster informing me that I needed to have a naked shower before I got into the pool, and highlighting the areas that I needed to wash. It made me laugh at first but then my courage almost failed me for a moment when I realised what it was asking of me. It was one thing to get to a place of acceptance of my new breast for myself; it was another to put my scarred and differently formed body on public display and I didn't know if I was ready to do that. I imagined women with fabulous bodies staring at mine, or children pointing and asking, 'What's that, mummy?'

And then I thought that this might be the only time in my life I would ever visit Iceland, the only chance I would get to swim in this particular pool. This is what I looked like now, and I did not want to treat my body as if it was something to be ashamed of. I surreptitiously stripped off, put my clothes in a locker and went for a shower before putting my swimming costume on. Of course no one even looked my way. It was strangely liberating and another step towards accepting my new normal. The pool was 50m long, in the open air with a huge spectator stand to one side that had seen better days, and a line of hot tubs underneath it of different temperatures, from hot to far too hot. Jonny and I swam, splashed, and soaked to our hearts' content.

Later in the week we drove to see thundering waterfalls and walked along dramatic beaches of black sand; we watched while geysers sent plumes of hot water into the air and sat in stunned silence at the edge of a frozen lake, overawed by its quiet beauty. We took our swimming stuff with us everywhere we went and tried out other pools as we came across them. I got blasé about stripping off in the changing rooms and by the end of the week I was doing it without further thought.

We drove to Gamla Laugin, the Secret Lagoon, Iceland's oldest swimming pool. It is dug out of the ground with a natural earth floor and surroundings, and decking along one edge to help people get in and out. Hot springs bubble out of the ground around the pool and run directly into it, producing clouds of steam that hang in the air like an over-enthusiastic smoke machine at a gig, adding an air of mystery to the atmosphere. We stayed in the hot water until our fingertips were wrinkled, watching the sun sink towards the horizon and catching snowflakes in our mouths as they gently tumbled into the water. It was magical.

Back home, I returned to work and took better care of myself. Choosing to be vulnerable with a few people who listened and helped me sort out my tangled thoughts meant that I was less afraid of falling apart in the office, and I could be a more competent version of myself there. Getting stuck in to solving problems and organising events reminded me of what I was good at and why I did that job in the first place. Catching the dark thoughts when they began to gather at the corners of my mind and gently probing them before they took root stopped me talking myself into despair. And I ran regularly.

For years, it had been my Sunday evening habit to look at the week ahead and work out when I could run, but now more than ever I made sure that I didn't go more than a couple of days without running. Just as the oncologist had prescribed me drugs to target the cancer, I prescribed myself running, treating it like a regular medication that I needed to keep me well. The 'runner's high' is much contested with different theories as to whether it really exists and what exactly causes it, but there is a clear link between running and better mental health.

Once again running gave me some much-needed headspace, a sense of competence and agency, and the simple healing effect of breathing deeply in the open air. Running had been so many things to me over the years. It started as a space to achieve and to expand my expectations of what I was capable of. It became an enjoyable way to stay fit and healthy, and to delight in my physical self. It was a source of great friendships and a community both to belong to and to contribute to. It was a way to express solidarity with people in Palestine and highlight their fundamental human rights.

Through my treatment it had been a vital link to my sense of identity, keeping me connected to who I really was when it felt that was all being stripped away. And now it was a therapeutic place and part of the healing process of coming back to myself. Slowly, intentionally, quietly I found my way towards more of a sense of equilibrium. My heart and soul were slowly catching up with my body in inhabiting my new normal.

It was time for another championship race. The Thames Towpath Ten is organised by West 4 Harriers, a neighbouring running club in Chiswick, and sponsored by the local brewery. There was a good turnout of Eagles, around 70 of us in total. The race starts with a couple of laps of a field to give the runners a bit of time to spread out and then heads over Chiswick Bridge and along the south side of the river past Kew Bridge and towards Richmond. It covered some of the same ground as my chemo runs and it was nice to be back there with a bit more energy and speed.

My running had been going well and so I set out to run 8:30 minute miles for a target finishing time of 1 hour 25. Trying to get my fitness back, I found that I was having to battle more than ever the internal monologue in a run that says this is too hard; I can't keep this up; I'm not going to make it. It had been more powerful over the previous few months because I didn't have any evidence to counteract it; I couldn't remind myself of previous PBs and races because they had all been achieved pre-cancer, and I needed to discover what I could achieve now.

During this race that internal tape was playing loud and clear but checking in with my body, I felt quite good. I started saying to myself 'strong and tall' as I ran, to drown out 'this is too hard', and found some people that were going at my pace that I could tuck in behind from time to time. I didn't have much in reserve for a sprint finish but I crossed the line just under 1 hour 24 minutes, very pleased with myself. A good race is not necessarily one where you run faster than you ever have before, but one where you win the mental battle so you are listening to your body and not the voice in your head, where you are intentional about how you run, strong and tall, and where you finish knowing that you have given it your best. I felt pleased that I had run a good race.

There was one more championship race to go – the Ealing Mile. A lap of Lammas Park in Ealing is, very conveniently, exactly one mile long and the Ealing Half-Marathon team hosted a regular mile race there on the first Friday of every month. I had done it a few times in the past and I have to say that the mile is my least-favourite distance. Send me out for a long marathon training run and I will come back in a few hours, exhausted but happy. Ask me to run as fast as I can for a few minutes in a mile race and normally I will find any number of excuses why I can't make it. I like to think that my body is better designed for long-distance running; I think the truth is that I just do not enjoy the chest-burning all-out effort that running fast requires.

However, this mile race was being organised by EHM just for our club championships and looking at the results spreadsheet, I worked out that if I came 18th or faster out of the women I would be third in my age category. So much for being happy just to take part and qualify, my competitive self was clearly alive and well and wanting some attention.

I had a meeting in Canterbury on the day of the race but I had managed to arrange it so that I could get back in time for the 7pm start. It was a productive meeting and I got caught up in everything that was happening down there. Afterwards I stayed behind to chat to the development worker about a grant application that he was intending to submit to my organisation and what extra information he could provide so it would fit the criteria better. Walking back to the station, I felt pleased with how it had all gone, especially after the time it had taken me to get my head back into work. That was until I checked the time of my train ticket and realised that I was going to miss the train that I needed to be on to get to Lammas Park in time. For some reason I had got my timings all wrong. Cue a frustrated half hour on the station platform, cursing my inattention and waiting for the next train to King's Cross.

From there I needed to get the tube to Ealing which would take another hour. As I sat on the train, I did some calculations and worked out that there was still a possibility of making the race if I went straight there from the tube station. I didn't have my running kit or trainers, but there was going to be a men's race and a women's race so I figured that I would be able to borrow some shoes and run in my work clothes. At King's Cross, I ran between the mainline platform and the underground, getting on the first tube train that arrived. I willed it to go faster, and once we were out in the open again I kept recalculating my arrival time on an app on my phone. It was touch and go as to whether I was going to make it.

I got to Acton Town, one stop away, and there was a change of driver which brought another couple of minutes' delay. That is when I remembered that I needed to be wearing an Eagles vest in order for the race to count towards the club championships and I didn't have one. In a parallel life, I persevered and ran from the tube to Lammas Park, getting there just in time. I borrowed some trainers and someone had a spare vest that I wore. I did even better than 18th place in the women's race and I got that third place in my age category. But in this life, my real life, my marred-by-cancer-but-getting-back-to-normal life I got off the train at Acton Town and got the one to Ealing Broadway that would take me home, to where Jonny was cooking supper and his sister Esther was staying the night.

At the end of my year of cancer treatment, I had said that I wouldn't set myself lots of running goals, that I would wait to see how the year unfolded, that I would run in beautiful places and savour every moment. Checking the app on my phone for the umpteenth time, I suddenly caught sight of myself. Here I was, a few months later, getting ridiculously stressed about, let's face it, an inconsequential championship placing and beating myself up over losing track of time.

I wanted running to be fun and life-enhancing, like my 50th parkrun had been, not a source of angst and self-criticism. And so I switched trains. There would be other races, other competitions, and other opportunities to see what I could do. Running had been so many different things to me and had given me so much. I was still working out what role it would play in my life post-cancer, but running was not my master and it was not the only thing that mattered. In that moment, a glass of wine and a meal in good company seemed much more sensible and inviting. Time to go home.

11

Back in Palestine

April

DURING those weeks of recovery, a friend who'd had treatment for cancer many years before said to me, 'Your next task is to get cancer from here' – pointing to her forehead – 'to here' – pointing to the back of her head. Slowly I found that it was shifting, from being the paradigm that framed all my thinking, from being the hum that I could not ignore when my mind was ticking idly over, to being something that had happened in the past and which occasionally I even forgot about.

When I had last been in Palestine a year before I knew I had a lump in my breast, but it had not dominated my thoughts. I only worried about it faintly in the odd moments when nothing much was going on, before telling myself that worrying did not achieve anything. Getting ready to go back made me think about just how much had happened in a year. It also gave me a welcome outward focus after months of self-preservation, of needing to be turned inwards on myself to cope with what was happening to me.

It was a motley crew that gathered at Luton airport early one morning to fly to Tel Aviv. There were 17 of us in Team Amos this year, ranging in age from 17 to 70, not many of us very experienced in the running game but all of us excited about the opportunity ahead. Eight people would be doing their first half-marathon, including Chris's son Jack who was the youngest on the team. Mike Sillitoe was there to do his 50th marathon, and Tracey Elliott was back to do the half again.

I had written training plans for a couple of people who had never run before and had enjoyed following their progress on Twitter as they went through the transition from 'I can't do this' to 'wow, I think I'm ready!' This time, we got through security without any hold-ups and were soon in a minibus on our way to Bethlehem.

There is something about Palestine that has captured my heart – the warmth of the people, the injustice of the situation, the beauty of the land. And I especially love being there for the marathon. There is something very normal and familiar about the mechanics of doing a race but in this setting it generates a disproportionate amount of joy. It was wonderful to be back, to see old friends and introduce new ones to the places I loved.

We spent the first day in Jerusalem, visiting sites that were familiar from Bible stories, and hearing from our guide about the challenges of living there. As the day wore on, I found myself getting rather disheartened. It felt like the situation is only getting worse. The settlements get inexorably bigger; land confiscations increase as border stones are moved and the wall encroaches; daily life continues to be disrupted and worn down; the stresses of living under occupation were taking their toll on some of my friends. But a phrase that is often used by Palestinians about the context they are living in is that they do not have the luxury of despair; they have to get on with life.

Chris had arranged for us to that afternoon meet a woman who works for Grassroots Jerusalem, a movement which encourages local people to network and bring about change for themselves. She was passionate and angry, so tired of talking about human rights and international law, of taking part in dialogue when the participants are so unequal, of expecting foreign governments to put pressure on Israel and bring change, of peace-building initiatives that create activity and generate funds for non-governmental organisations but not Palestinian organisations.

That anger and passion are driving her to build something positive, to get local groups articulating their vision for Jerusalem, to imagine and co-create a different way of living that prepares for a time when there will be peace. Her work is to enable Palestinians to take the initiative themselves rather than expecting other people to bring about change and asks the question, 'What does the day after the occupation look like, in your organisation, your community, your city?'

I think some people in our group wanted to persuade her that dialogue is always worthwhile, that international law is crucial. And I think I would agree with them. But I loved how she had found her calling and agency, her distinctive contribution to bringing change in this complex situation. I found myself thinking that this is what all of us need to discover, in whatever mess we find ourselves, the unique contribution we can make to bring about change, and the energy and passion to get on and do it.

She talked about the people she meets who give her hope, who find ways to work together to counteract the challenges of the occupation. Listening to her, I thought how giving in to despair leads you into a dead end, there is nowhere else to go, whereas doing something constructive about the situation you are in provides a space to imagine a different future and for hope to grow.

We went to collect our race numbers from the Peace Centre in Manger Square. Each year the organisation of the race gets slicker, but the sense of excitement among both participants and organisers does not diminish. Volunteers welcomed us with huge smiles and asked us where we were from. We checked that our envelopes held our timing chips and enough safety pins and had our photos taken holding our race numbers and shirts in front of a banner, rituals that will be familiar to anyone who has taken part in a race like this. I could see the apprehension on the faces of those in our team who were doing their first half-marathon; it suddenly all seemed very real now.

We walked through Bethlehem to Aida Refugee Camp where I had met Mohammed on my first visit to Palestine. I wondered what he was doing now, four years on. We went to Alrowwad, a performing arts organisation that works with children and young people to encourage what they call 'beautiful resistance', empowering them to make a positive difference to their community in non-violent ways.

Chris was working with Abdelfattah Abusrour, its founder, to try and bring a group of young people from Alrowwad to the UK that summer. The plan was for them to perform at the Edinburgh Festival and various other places and to give the young people a taste of life outside a refugee camp, to meet their peers over here who have never experienced tear gas or walls or restrictions on their movement. It was a huge undertaking to get everything lined up, including the visas they would need to travel, but meeting the teenagers who were looking forward to the trip made Chris even more determined to make it happen.

They danced and sang for us, their infectious energy and smiles getting our feet tapping and hands clapping along in rhythm. At the end they pulled us to our feet and showed us how to do their traditional dance, Dabke. Where they had been leaping in the air moments before, we shuffled and tripped over our feet but they patiently showed us again and again until we managed a passable Dabke line dance. They graciously applauded us and promised to come and watch us run.

The next morning we gathered with hordes of other runners in Manger Square. It was mildly chaotic as usual with taxis driving right into the square to drop people off even though it was meant to be traffic-free, and most people ignoring the barriers that were supposed to separate the runners into the different distances they were doing.

There are very few portaloos in Palestine so local restaurants had been persuaded to let runners use their facilities. I joined the queue in a café where we had drunk mint lemonade the day before. I got talking to a woman who works for the UN in Gaza, and who was there to run the marathon. She told me that, at the last minute, over 100 athletes in Gaza had found out that they had not got permission to travel to Bethlehem to take part in the race, including Nader al-Masri who had won it the year before, and 15-year-old Inas Nofal, Gaza's only female competitive runner. It was the only cloud over the race, frustrating but sadly unsurprising.

I met up with Su and Helen, and got choked up thinking about what connected the three of us. And then someone introduced me to Philippa Whitford, a Scottish MP. The race warm-up was happening just behind us with dance music blaring out of the loudspeakers so it was hard to have a decent conversation but I discovered that she had been a breast cancer surgeon for many years before joining parliament in the election the year before. She had volunteered in Al-Ahli Hospital 25 years earlier, and she was staying in Bethlehem for a couple of days on her way to Gaza, to spend her parliamentary recess back at the hospital.

British MPs had not been allowed into the Gaza Strip since 2009, and she was travelling in her identity as a surgeon, hoping that they would not ask too many questions about what else she did. She said, 'If they Google me, I'm stuffed!'

We heard later that she had been allowed in and had performed four major operations on women with breast cancer, as well as leading seminars and assessing breast cancer provision right across Palestine. Meeting her just before the race started was inspirational, a reminder of why I was running and what I was raising money for. For months, I had been aware that women in Gaza were not getting the treatment they needed for breast cancer and it felt serendipitous to meet Philippa just before we ran, someone who could make such a practical and much-needed contribution, someone who would be listened to when she got back home.

It was time to line up at the start in a nervous crowd of marathon and half-marathon runners. And then we were off, running through the streets that we had explored on foot over the last few days, heading out on what was now a very familiar route for me, along the wall, through Aida refugee camp and out on the road towards Hebron. We ran past a shepherd herding his sheep along the side of the road, nervous animals eyeing these strange runners. We ran past children hanging out of the windows of their houses to laugh at us and cheer us on. We ran past people who really did not care that a race was happening and who just wanted to get on with their normal everyday life.

I had a target in my head, to finish in under two hours like at Wokingham, and it took me a while to settle into a regular pace. It was an emotional run for me, thinking about all that had happened since I was last here. I had experienced fear, loneliness, illness, pain and despair like never before, but also deep friendship, compassion, care and inspiration. People I had never met before had used their skills to save my life and coax me back to health. Family and friends had stepped into the strange space I found myself in and had shown their love for me in practical and sacrificial ways. I found myself saying thank you as I ran, to the rhythm of my feet pounding on the road, wanting this experience to count for something, and for my run to be a prayer of gratitude.

Heading back to Manger Square, the road was full of people doing the 10k, who had set off after us but who were now happily walking the distance. I wove in and out of them, and slowed to a walk every so often. I crossed the finish line in just over two hours, missing my target by 25 seconds, another finishing time to add to the many over the years that ended up on the wrong side of what I had originally intended.

There was a confusing crowd of people bunching up just beyond the finishing line to hand in their timing chips and grab their medals. I put my timing chip in the top pocket of someone who looked official, hoping that it would end up in the right place, and joined Chris and Jack at the finish. We took photos and cheered other members of Team Amos as they crossed the line, sharing in the delight of those who had just done their first half-marathon. We watched Brian, the oldest member of our team, and Mike head out for their second lap to do the full marathon and then went to have showers, feeling faintly guilty that we were getting clean and cool while they still were out in the hot sun.

Back at the finish line, we ate falafel wraps for lunch and waited for Mike and Brian. By now the town was getting back to normal with cars on the route and men lining up in the square for Friday prayers. Mike finished in just under five hours, and we knew from Brian's half-marathon time that he would probably take six hours or longer. The awards ceremony had taken place and the number of people waiting around dwindled as the race organisers started to pack things away. The cut-off time for the race was six hours, and we stood nervously at the top of the hill by the finishing line looking out for a sighting of Brian at the bottom. We found out afterwards that about three miles before the end, the police told him that he needed to stop running because of tear gas ahead.

The marathon route goes past an Israeli watchtower set in the wall about a mile and a half from the end. For several Fridays there had been demonstrations there with tear gas fired by the soldiers, and this Friday was no exception. Six times the police asked him to get in their car, and six times he refused because he wanted to finish his marathon. Eventually, the police drove the race organisers out to meet him and a couple of other runners who were still on the course. They persuaded them to get in a car and have a short lift past the worst of the tear gas.

Brian agreed but once they were safely past the site of the demonstration, he got out and started running again. For the last couple of miles he had his own personal police escort with a motorbike in front and a car behind. It was a great moment when we saw him appear at the bottom of the hill, and we cheered like mad as he made it to the top. Lia, his partner, was there to greet him with a huge hug, and then it became clear why he was so determined to finish the race. He produced a ring out of the pocket of his shorts and got down on one knee to propose to Lia. She gave him an ecstatic 'yes', while we all took photos and hugged them in delight. They became local celebrities for the rest of our time in Bethlehem as the story spread. Everyone loves a wedding.

On our final day in Palestine, we went to Al-Arroub refugee

camp, about ten miles outside Bethlehem. On our trip the year before, we had visited a plot just outside the camp, set in a beautiful valley of fields and olive groves. Back then the plot had been a tangle of twisted wire and concrete rubble. We met the family who owned the land and heard how they had been building their house there for four years, only for it to be demolished one day before they had had a chance to even live in it. Since then they had been squashed into a tiny flat deep inside the camp, their only option of somewhere to live. It was not just their house that had been destroyed; it was their hopes and dreams for their future, their ability to raise their children in the way they would choose and to put down roots in a community.

Shortly after that, Amos had taken a team of volunteers over to rebuild their house, in an act of solidarity and as a very practical protest at the demolitions taking place. This year it was hard to believe that it was the same place. Instead of climbing over rubble and feeling a sense of despair, we were proudly invited into a beautiful new home, not quite finished but with ample space for the family to spread out, to feel safer and to get on with their lives. They offered us cups of sage tea, and found us all places to sit, delighted to be able to offer us hospitality in return for the gift that had been given to them. Look how much can change in just one year.

Usually when I get home after finishing a race, I stuff the medal into a box in my study alongside all the others I have collected over the years. They are a nice memento to have but I don't feel the need to keep them on display. The olive wood medals from my races in Palestine are different; they hang from a shelf above my desk, a reminder of the race, the place and the people I have met. Back home, I hung this year's medal beside the other three and took a moment to reflect:

This is for the Gazan athletes who didn't get permission to travel to Bethlehem and had to miss the race after months of training;

This is for the teenagers in Aida Camp who danced their hearts out for us while we were there;

This is for all the people we met who are working for a different future for this beautiful country;

This is for Team Amos who exceeded their expectations by running for justice and peace;

This is for the women of Gaza who deserve far better care for what should be a treatable disease;

And this is for Liz, Alice, Helen, Su Mac and me, all of us hit by this thing called breast cancer; all of us have run one hell of a race.

12

Living Hopefully

THERE are so many of us. Those who find a lump and with it the relentless worry about what it might mean. Those who sit in front of a consultant with fear in their hearts and hear the words, 'I'm sorry, it is cancer.' Those who then have to pass that on to the people they love, knowing that the words they are about to say will spread that fear and pain, 'I'm afraid it is cancer.' Those who will always wonder what they could have done to avoid getting to that place. Those for whom life will never be the same again.

I know that I am fortunate. The cancer was found early enough that it was caught before it had spread too far. I was given the treatment I needed straight away. I had family and friends who stepped into the strange world of that cancer diagnosis and who kept me company, gave me courage and cheered me on. I had running to help me hold on to my identity and give me something to focus on through the long months of treatment. But I know that I would be in a better place if I had acted earlier. And there is always the possibility that it will return.

I had a conversation with a church leader just before Christmas. He asked if my surgery had been successful, 'Are you now cancer-free?' I said, 'Yes, hopefully.' He did not like that. 'No, be positive! You can do it!' As if all that stands between me and a long and healthy future is my attitude of mind. As if being honest about doubts and fears will cause them to become a reality. As if it will be my fault somehow if the cancer recurs. I don't subscribe to that point of view.

Anyone who has treatment for cancer lives with the knowledge that it might return. As I have said, there is no going back to the sweet oblivion of when cancer was something that happened to other people. I don't want to ignore what has happened to me and live in denial that it could happen again. But nor do I want to treat what is only a possibility as if it was a certainty, and live under the shadow of something that actually may not happen.

I know the stats that tell me how many women with the same diagnosis as me were alive five years or ten years later but of course I don't know which side of the percentage I will end up on, in the nice big majority or on the smaller but deadlier side. And living hopefully seems to me to be the best approach to have.

In her book, *Men Explain Things To Me*, Rebecca Solnit has an essay about the possibility of bringing about change, of people and movements shaping history, of how living with uncertainty and doubt can open up new possibilities. She quotes Virginia Woolf, 'The future is dark which is the best thing the future can be, I think.'

And she then goes on to say, 'To me, the grounds for hope are simply that we don't know what will happen next, and that the unlikely and unimaginable transpire quite regularly... Despair is a form of certainty, certainty that the future will be a lot like the present or will decline from it; despair is a confident memory of the future. Optimism is similarly confident about what will happen. Both are grounds for not acting. Hope can be the knowledge that we don't have that memory and that reality doesn't necessarily match our plans.'

Although she is writing about a different context, her words resonate with me. My reality over the last year has not matched the plans I made. I feel I've been cracked open; the assumptions that I made about my life have been shattered. I've been left more vulnerable and less certain, but also less alone and more loved. I don't know what will happen next but the darkness of the future, the lack of a script gives me grounds for hope. To be hopeful is to be expectant, to imagine the best outcome, while also living with the reality that anything could happen. Hope lives in that space between despair and optimism, and looks for what is emerging.

Training for a race is an exercise in hopefulness. You sign up with a goal in mind, perhaps to run faster than ever before, or to try a different distance, or as an excuse to visit a new city. You commit yourself to a training plan and carve out time so you can follow it. You drink less wine and eat more healthily, wanting to give your body the best chance of success. But you don't know what will happen next.

There will be times when everything aligns and you run the perfect race. There will be times when you get injured and you have to modify your expectations of what you can achieve. There will be times when you have to give up on the race, take time to heal and start again in a few weeks' time. But it all starts with the choice to act hopefully.

There is no going back once you have had cancer. There is no knowing what the future holds, but you do have a choice about how you will move forward. I will do what I can to live well and to live healthily but ultimately I cannot control what happens next. And that is quite liberating; it is not down to me. I will keep my hope, thank you very much. I choose to live hopefully.

Acknowledgements

WRITING a book is a strange mixture of creativity, hard graft, excitement, doubt, inspiration and dogged perseverance. It is a solitary task that draws you into a tunnel of writing, but it can only happen because of the multitude of people who contribute to the story you want to tell. I'm going to take this opportunity to thank everyone who has played a part in this book in one way or another by joining me in my experience of cancer – what amazing people you are.

Thank you to everyone at Pitch Publishing for enabling this book to happen.

Thank you to the medical teams at Ealing and Charing Cross Hospitals, especially Ms Shah, Dr Lewanski, Jude Hunter, Nikki Kettley and Makaita Kakomwe. It is no easy task to take frightened and grieving people through treatment for cancer and I'm so grateful for your expertise, wisdom and kindness.

A huge thank you to my chemo runners, Lucy Rigg, Harry Baker, Christine Elliott, Mandy Keasley, Liz Low, Joel Baker and Neil Enskat. I don't know if you realised quite what you were doing for me at the time, but it made such a difference.

Thank you to Mary Slark, John and Meg Payne, Susie, Dave, Carrie and Jake Stanforth, Jan and Greg Watson for walking with me on the day of my last treatment and for all your love throughout it.

Thank you to Ealing Eagles Running Club for being the catalyst that has made me run further and faster, and for being such a remarkable community. Thank you to all the many Eagles who drew alongside me in different ways last year – a special mention for Kelvin Walker, Mark and Anthea Yabsley, Godfrey Rust, Tracey Melville, Katie Murray, Lou Plank and Richard Tucson.

Thank you to everyone else who pops up in these pages for being part of the story – to Maggi Dawn, Azariah and Anna France-Williams, Bethany Eckley, Bianca, Becca Dean, Jon and Clare Birch, Julie Johnson, Lowell Sheppard, Chris Wheelwright, Sheenagh and Richard Burrell.

Thank you to Chris Rose, the incredible team at Amos Trust and to everyone who has come to run in Palestine. See you there next year.

Thank you to the Baker clan for keeping me going, to Susie and Steve, Dave and Lou, Ruth and Derek for your generosity and gentle concern, to Alison and Esther for the prayers I couldn't pray for myself.

Thank you to my wonderful work colleagues who gave me unwavering support and did my job as well as their own.

A salute to Liz O'Riordan, Alice-May Purkiss, Su McClellan and Helen Powell whose experiences of breast cancer mingled with mine in different ways. I'm honoured to have such strong and gorgeous women as my friends.

Thank you to Jan Leach, Claire Angus, Sara Cunningham, Signe Gosmann, Melanie Aram and Emily Hughes for getting me through that exam and for your love and friendship.

Thank you to Rachel Hodson for keeping me running over so many years through your chiropractic genius.

Thank you to everyone who commented on my blog, interacted with me on social media, and who sent me cards, flowers and gifts. I felt seen and held and loved.

Thank you to those who read drafts of this book and made suggestions for how it could be improved: Lucy Rigg, Christine Elliott, Julia Wickham, Jane Walker and Jonny Baker.

I've told my story through the lens of running and so there are people who made a huge difference to me while I was having treatment but who aren't in the book because, in spite of knowing me for many years, they are not runners.

They deserve a mention here. Thank you to: Julia Wickham for deep friendship and for your goodbye the night before my surgery; Wendy Beech Ward for your compassion and the faithful phone calls to see how I was; Anna Poulson for always seeing the beauty in brokenness; Sonia Mainstone Cotton for your cards and gifts that started arriving before my treatment and kept coming until after it had finished; Mike and Jill Rose for fabulous and undemanding meals, for letting me fall asleep on your sofa, and for making sure that Jonny was okay.

Thank you to Joel, Kat, Flo, Harry and Grace for everything. You are my reason for living hopefully.

Thank you to Jonny for doing all this with me – for midwinter parkruns, for sourdough bread, for being my safe space, for loving me. I want to grow old with you.

Permissions

Permission to use the translation of *The Guesthouse* by Rumi has been kindly granted by Coleman Barks. Quotes from *Late Fragments* by Kate Gross are reprinted by permission of HarperCollins Publishers Ltd © Kate Gross 2015. Included with the kind permission of Lizzy Hawker and Aurum Press, quotation taken from *Runner: A Short Story About a Long Run* (2015). Permission to use transcribed quotes from Radio 4's Desert Island Discs interview with Lemn Sissay has been kindly given by Lemn Sissay and Radio 4. Quote from Victoria Pendleton in Donald McRae's article in The Guardian on 03/12/2015 used courtesy of Guardian News and Media Ltd. Quote from *Men Explain Things to Me* by Rebecca Solnit used with permission of Granta Books.